Department of Veterans Affairs
Health Services Research & Development Service | Evidence-based Synthesis Program

A Critical Review of the Literature Regarding Homelessness among Veterans

April 2011

Prepared for:
Department of Veterans Affairs
Veterans Health Administration
Health Services Research & Development Service
Washington, DC 20420

Prepared by:
Evidence-based Synthesis Program (ESP) Center
Portland VA Medical Center
Portland, OR
Devan Kansagara, MD, MCR, Director

Investigators:
(all authors contributed equally to this report):
Howard Balshem, MS
Vivian Christensen, PhD
Anais Tuepker, PhD

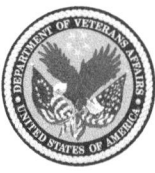

PREFACE

Health Services Research & Development Service's (HSR&D's) Evidence-based Synthesis Program (ESP) was established to provide timely and accurate syntheses of targeted healthcare topics of particular importance to Veterans Affairs (VA) managers and policymakers, as they work to improve the health and healthcare of Veterans. The ESP disseminates these reports throughout VA.

HSR&D provides funding for four ESP Centers and each Center has an active VA affiliation. The ESP Centers generate evidence syntheses on important clinical practice topics, and these reports help:

- develop clinical policies informed by evidence,
- guide the implementation of effective services to improve patient outcomes and to support VA clinical practice guidelines and performance measures, and
- set the direction for future research to address gaps in clinical knowledge.

In 2009, the ESP Coordinating Center was created to expand the capacity of HSR&D Central Office and the four ESP sites by developing and maintaining program processes. In addition, the Center established a Steering Committee comprised of HSR&D field-based investigators, VA Patient Care Services, Office of Quality and Performance, and Veterans Integrated Service Networks (VISN) Clinical Management Officers. The Steering Committee provides program oversight, guides strategic planning, coordinates dissemination activities, and develops collaborations with VA leadership to identify new ESP topics of importance to Veterans and the VA healthcare system.

Comments on this evidence report are welcome and can be sent to Nicole Floyd, ESP Coordinating Center Program Manager, at nicole.floyd@va.gov.

Recommend citation: Balshem H, Christensen V, Tuepker A, Kansagara D. A Critical Review of the Literature Regarding Homelessness among Veterans. VA-ESP Project #05-225: 2011

> This report is based on research conducted by the Evidence-based Synthesis Program (ESP) Center located at the Portland VA Medical Center, Portland, OR funded by the Department of Veterans Affairs, Veterans Health Administration, Office of Research and Development, Health Services Research and Development. The findings and conclusions in this document are those of the author(s) who are responsible for its contents; the findings and conclusions do not necessarily represent the views of the Department of Veterans Affairs or the United States government. Therefore, no statement in this article should be construed as an official position of the Department of Veterans Affairs. No investigators have any affiliations or financial involvement (e.g., employment, consultancies, honoraria, stock ownership or options, expert testimony, grants or patents received or pending, or royalties) that conflict with material presented in the report.

TABLE OF CONTENTS

EXECUTIVE SUMMARY
Background 1
Methods 1
Data Synthesis 2
Peer Review 2
Results 2
Limitations of the Evidence 5
Future Research 5
Abbreviations Table 7

INTRODUCTION
Background 9

METHODS
Topic Development 11
Search Strategy 11
Study Selection 12
Data Synthesis 12
Conceptual Model 12
Peer Review 13

RESULTS
Definitions of Homelessness 15
Assessing the Limitations of the Current Research 15
Data Sources 18
Methodological Considerations 21
Key Question #1a. What is the prevalence and incidence of homelessness among Veterans? ... 22
Key Question #1b. How has the prevalence and incidence of homelessness among Veterans changed over time? 23
Key Question #1c. How prevalent are psychiatric illness, substance abuse, and chronic medical illness among homeless Veterans? 23
Key Question #2a. Which risk factors are associated with new homelessness or a return to homelessness among Veterans? How do these risk factors differ from non-Veteran populations? 25
Key Question #2b. Have risk factors for homelessness among Veterans changed over time? ... 26
Key Question #3. Are there factors specific to military service that increase the risk of homelessness, or is the increased risk a marker for pre-military comorbidities and social support deficiencies? 26
Key Question #4. What is the relationship between incarceration and homelessness among Veterans? 34

SUMMARY AND DISCUSSION 41

    Recommendations for Future Research... 42

REFERENCES 44

FIGURES

    Figure 1. Risk Factors for Veteran Homelessness: Conceptual Model 14

APPENDIX A.   PEER REVIEW COMMENTS/AUTHOR RESPONSES 53

APPENDIX B.   TECHNICAL EXPERTS CONSULTED AND REVIEWERS 59

EXECUTIVE SUMMARY

BACKGROUND

In 2009, President Obama and Secretary Shinseki committed to ending homelessness among Veterans. In support of that effort, the Federal Strategic Plan to Prevent and End Homelessness 2010 developed by the United States Interagency Council on Homelessness (USICH) established as one of its goals to prevent and end homelessness among Veterans in five years. An understanding of the epidemiology of homelessness among Veterans and the methodological strengths and weaknesses of this evidence base may inform program-planning efforts and future research needs. Understanding the risk factors for homelessness among Veterans and how these risk factors compare to the general population is important in developing identification and prevention programs for Veterans at risk for homelessness. This report was requested by VA Central Office and The National Center for Homelessness Among Veterans as part of that effort to identify what is known and what is not known about the prevalence of homelessness among Veterans, and about the risk factors for homelessness among Veterans, including risk factors related to military service and incarceration.

The key questions were:

Key Questions #1a. What is the prevalence and incidence of homelessness among Veterans?

#1b. How has the prevalence and incidence of homelessness among Veterans changed over time?

#1c. How prevalent are psychiatric illness, substance abuse, and chronic medical illness among homeless Veterans?

Key Questions #2a. Which risk factors are associated with new homelessness or a return to homelessness among Veterans? How do these risk factors differ from non-Veteran populations?

#2b. Have risk factors for homelessness among Veterans changed over time?

Key Question #3. Are there factors specific to military service that increase the risk of homelessness, or is the increased risk a marker for pre-military comorbidities and social support deficiencies?

Key Question #4. What is the relationship between incarceration and homelessness among Veterans?

METHODS

Key questions were developed with the input of experts from the National Center for Homelessness Among Veterans and the VA New England Healthcare System, and with feedback from national experts on homelessness and homelessness among Veterans. A search for relevant literature was conducted in MEDLINE, the Cochrane Database of Systematic Reviews, Sociological Abstracts, and Criminal Justice Abstracts from database inception through

July 2010. We also monitored Table of Contents alerts for several publications to identify new research published in 2010; searched several non-medical qualitative journals including Qualitative Research and Qualitative Health Research; and sought guidance on other sources from a survey of technical experts. For all Key Questions, the reference lists of articles returned were reviewed for any additional relevant studies. Because of the exploratory nature of this review, few restrictions were placed on articles to be considered for inclusion.

DATA SYNTHESIS

The existing evidence base relevant to this topic does not lend itself to a quantitative synthesis, since sample populations and variables investigated were rarely consistent across studies. In this report, we did not conduct a quantitative data synthesis or meta-analysis, but rather focused on presenting the strength of each existing study's findings and developing a conceptual model for understanding what these findings mean collectively, as well as indicating where there are significant gaps in our knowledge on this topic.

PEER REVIEW

A draft version of this report was reviewed by six technical experts. Reviewer comments were addressed and our responses were incorporated in the final report (Appendix A).

RESULTS

KEY QUESTION #1A. What is the prevalence and incidence of homelessness among Veterans?

The recently released report *Veteran Homelessness: A Supplemental Report to the 2009 Annual Homeless Assessment Report to Congress* (2009 Veteran AHAR) estimates that on a single night in January 2009 there were 75,609 homeless Veterans and that an estimated 136,334 Veterans spent at least one night in an emergency shelter or transitional housing program between October 1, 2008 and September 30, 2009. With nearly 23 million Veterans in the U.S. population in 2009, the prevalence of Veterans experiencing homelessness on a single night in January 2009 was approximately 33 for every 10,000 Veterans. Approximately 60 out of every 10,000 Veterans spent at least one night in an emergency shelter or transitional housing between October 1, 2008 and September 30, 2009.

KEY QUESTION #1B. How has the prevalence and incidence of homelessness among Veterans changed over time?

Because of changes in reporting and in the methods for counting the number of homeless, estimates of the prevalence of homelessness among Veterans over time are not comparable. With regard to the percentage of Veterans among the homeless, in 1996, the National Survey of Homeless Assistance Providers and Clients estimated that 23 percent of the homeless population were Veterans. More recently, the first four Annual Homeless Assessment Reports (AHARs) estimated that the percentage of Veterans among the homeless stayed relatively steady at about 15 percent. The most recent AHAR reported a decrease to 16 percent of adults and 12 percent of all homeless individuals. The demographic composition of the Veteran homeless population is changing. According to the CHALENG report, VA facilities have recently reported an increase of 24 percent in homeless Veteran families seeking services. In addition, the percentage of homeless women Veterans is expected to increase as the percentage of female Veterans has increased dramatically in recent years.

KEY QUESTION #1C. How prevalent are psychiatric illness, substance abuse, and chronic medical illness among homeless Veterans?

There are few studies directly assessing the prevalence of psychiatric illness, substance abuse, or chronic illness in the general population of homeless Veterans. The 2009 Veteran AHAR estimates that approximately 53 percent of homeless Veterans have some kind of disability. This estimate is based on a definition of disability that includes substance abuse, mental illness, and physical disabilities. Estimates for specific disabilities are not provided. However, most other studies rely on already morbid populations seeking treatment for services and so cannot provide estimates of prevalence in the homeless population as a whole. Prevalence estimates from a limited evidence base vary. A study based on a convenience sample of homeless adults admitted to homeless shelters in Santa Clara County, California between November 1989 and March 1990 found that 17 percent of Veterans had been admitted for overnight treatment of psychiatric problems; that 29 percent reported actual and 39 percent perceived alcohol abuse; and 22 percent reported illegal drug use. More recently, a survey of randomly selected homeless adults in Pittsburgh and Philadelphia found that 61.4 percent reported psychiatric problems, 79.5 percent reported alcohol or drug abuse or dependence, and 66.1 percent reported having at least one chronic medical condition.

KEY QUESTION #2A. Which risk factors are associated with new homelessness or a return to homelessness among Veterans? How do these risk factors differ from non-Veteran populations?

Risk factors most strongly and consistently associated with homelessness in both Veteran and non-Veteran populations include childhood risk factors such as inadequate care by the parents, experiencing foster care or group placement, and prolonged periods of running away from home. Low or unstable income, low social support and a history of incarceration appear to place both Veterans and non-Veterans at increased risk for homelessness.

The most important risk factors for homelessness do not differ substantially between Veteran and non-Veteran populations. There are notable differences in the prevalence of some characteristics often found to be protective: Veteran homeless tend to be older and better educated; to have had better, early family cohesion; and are more likely to be or have been married than non-Veteran homeless. The reasons for this lack of expected protection are not well understood. It may be that the differences between these populations are too small to influence outcomes significantly. Alternatively, there may be unique Veteran experiences associated with either service or post-deployment readjustment that actively undermine the protective mechanism associated with these factors in other populations.

KEY QUESTION #2B. Have risk factors for homelessness among Veterans changed over time?

Evidence shows that over time, certain risk factors become more salient than others and affect different sub-populations. With the increasing number of women in the military, military sexual trauma (MST) has become an important and prevalent additional trauma-associated risk factor. The wars in Iraq and Afghanistan have led to an increase in the number of National Guard Veterans serving often repeated tours of duty in these conflicts. Since these Veterans are more likely to have families during and immediately after deployment, the importance of factors related to homelessness among families may increase. Economic and structural factors also strongly influence who is at risk. In good economic times, those most vulnerable because of personal risk factors will become homeless; as economic conditions worsen, an increasing number of those less vulnerable will also become homeless.

KEY QUESTION #3. Are there factors specific to military service that increase the risk of homelessness, or is the increased risk a marker for pre-military comorbidities and social support deficiencies?

Some studies have found that homeless Veterans have lower prevalence of some general population risk factors (such as family dysfunction) and higher prevalence of protective factors (such as higher educational levels). These findings suggest that pre-military risk factors or comorbidities do not account for the over-representation of Veterans among the nation's homeless. Veterans appear to be at risk for homelessness for much the same reasons as other Americans. However, their unique experiences as Veterans may mean that the pathways through which they come to be exposed to or develop these risks may be qualitatively different. This is an area which warrants further research.

An example of the influence of unique Veteran experiences may be found in considering the existing evidence on the impact of combat exposure. Although associated with only a subset of Veterans and homeless Veterans, prolonged or intense combat exposure has been found to negatively impact mental health, employment, income and social support, thus indirectly but substantially increasing the risk of homelessness among those Veterans who have had intense combat exposure compared to those who have not. Given that non-Veterans in the United States are unlikely to experience intense combat exposure, their pathways to low social support or poor mental health can only partially inform our understanding of homelessness among Veterans.

Some behaviors which may place Veterans at increased risk of homelessness seem likely to emerge during military service or during the readjustment/post-deployment period. These include problem alcohol use, problem substance use and/or low social support. While exposure to these risk factors is not intrinsic to military service, evidence suggests that military culture and/or the inherently disruptive nature of military service tours increase the likelihood of negative outcomes for both substance use and social support.

Though only examined to date by one small study, MST has been associated with increased risk of homelessness among female Veterans. Further research is needed.

KEY QUESTION #4. What is the relationship between incarceration and homelessness among Veterans?

After a steady rise in the number of Veterans in prison since 1985, the number, which peaked at about 153,100 in 2000, had declined by about 9 percent to 140,000 by 2004. Literature on incarceration and homelessness makes apparent the demographic similarities between homeless and incarcerated populations – both are typically poor, uneducated, and minority populations with few job skills – and suggests a bi-directional association between homelessness and incarceration. Factors found to be associated with homelessness among the incarcerated include ineffective discharge planning, legal and regulatory restrictions, full sentencing laws, and financial instability.

LIMITATIONS OF THE EVIDENCE

Although there is consistent evidence associating specific risk factors such as substance abuse and mental illness with homelessness, there are significant limitations with the data in terms of how well risk factors were defined and prevalence measured. Association does not, on its own, indicate causality, and very few studies reviewed were designed to measure the direction of associations. Studies are limited by several factors, including: inclusion of morbid populations seen in clinical settings that may not be generalizable to the broader population of Veterans; use of varying and often inconsistent definitions of homelessness; use of measures of unproven validity; and limitations in study design.

FUTURE RESEARCH

This report identifies a number of gaps in the literature and makes key suggestions to define an agenda for future research on Veteran homelessness:

- Longitudinal studies with Operation Enduring Freedom (OEF)/Operation Iraqi Freedom (OIF) Veterans are needed to capture data on exposures occurring before homelessness occurs. Given the VA's current policy of pro-active enrollment and engagement of this cohort, opportunities exist to conduct longitudinal studies that collect information on all of the risk factors identified in this report. This research should control for structural risk factors such as housing market costs and available assistance programs.

- Longitudinal studies with all new cohorts of enlisting military service members could better determine the pre-existing presence of risk factors such as low social support, alcohol or substance abuse problems before military service. Policies should be developed to facilitate the use of data from enlistment screenings in research.

- Qualitative studies employing longitudinal, ethnographic methods to investigate the distinct experiences of homeless Veterans will help researchers to understand what is unique about Veteran exposure to risk factors common to the general homeless population. This remains poorly understood at present but may have important implications for designing homelessness prevention programs that will be effective for Veterans.

- Current research suggests that risk for violent criminal behavior varies by service branch. Research to confirm these differences and how to identify individuals at risk for continued post-military violent criminal behavior may help target interventions to those most at risk for post-military incarceration.

- Research on the post-deployment period is needed, with a particular focus on risk factors for loss of income and social support during this transition period, as well as rates of short-term homelessness experienced during this period. These data could be collected as part of longitudinal studies looking for relationships between short-term and more chronic homelessness, a topic that has been the focus of past research.

- Further research on MST, its relationship to homelessness, and appropriate MST prevention and treatment programs is recommended.

- Research on Veterans Courts and other types of specialty courts should be conducted in order to determine how they can most effectively provide alternatives to incarceration for Veterans.

- Systems-perspective research on collaborations among Departments of Corrections, the VA, the Department of Housing and Urban Development (HUD), and local community health agencies could inform efforts to reduce the likelihood of homelessness upon re-entry from incarceration, including developing a better understanding of how to identify those most at risk for homelessness post-release.

- Most of the measures used to assess risk factors and personal characteristics of the homeless, including measures of substance abuse, mental health, and measures of social support, have been developed and normed on populations living in conditions very different from the homeless. The applicability of these measures to homeless populations is unknown. Research should be undertaken to assess the applicability of these measures, and to modify or develop new measures where warranted. Similarly, better defined research on the aspects of social support most relevant to improving Veterans' post-deployment adjustment would contribute both to addressing Veteran homelessness and the literature's broader understanding of the function of social support.

- Long-term studies repeatedly collecting both quantitative and qualitative data, though always relatively difficult and costly to conduct, would greatly improve our understanding of Veterans' difficulties in re-engagement and re-integration over long periods of time after deployment, not just in the initial post-deployment year, which is more frequently studied.

- Studies that include both individual and structural risk factors should be conducted to assess both their independent and contingent effects.

- Research is needed to investigate the relationship between the unique Veteran experience of "family readjustment difficulties" in the post-deployment period and other, more generalized concepts such as social support, as well as the relationship between family readjustment difficulties and clinical diagnoses of mental illness.

- To our knowledge, the direct relationship between injury/disability and increased risk of homelessness has not been well studied in the Veteran population. There is a need for research designed to examine injury as a risk factor for homelessness, both directly and indirectly, and taking into account the complex effects of serious injury on both income and quality of life/well-being.

ABBREVIATIONS TABLE

ACCESS	Access to Community Care and Effective Service Supports
AFDC	Aid to Families with Dependent Children
AHAR	Annual Homeless Assessment Report
ASI	Addiction Severity Index
CHALENG	Community Homelessness Assessment, Local Education and Networking Group
CI	Confidence interval
CMHS	Center for Mental Health Services
CoC	Continuum of Care
DCHV	Domiciliary Care for Homeless Veterans
DRRI	Deployment Risk and Resilience Inventory
DSM-IV	Diagnostic and Statistical Manual of Mental Disorders, Fourth Edition
ELI	Extremely Low Income
ESP	Evidence-based Synthesis Program
FMR	Fair market rent
GAINS	National GAINS Center: Gathering information; Assessing what works; Interpreting/integrating the facts; Networking; Stimulating change
GAO	Government Accounting Office
HCHV	Health Care for Homeless Veterans
HCMI	Homeless Chronically Mentally Ill Veterans Program
Health VIEWS	Health of Vietnam Era Veteran Women's Study
HEARTH	Homeless Emergency and Rapid Transition to Housing
HMIS	Homeless Management Information System
HR	Hazard ratio
HSR&D	Health Services Research and Development Service
HUD	Department of Housing and Urban Development
MCS	Millennium Cohort Study
MOS	Medical Outcomes Study
MPSI	Multi-Problem Screening Inventory
MST	Military sexual trauma
N or n	Number
NSHAPC	National Survey of Homeless Assistance Providers and Clients
NVVRS	National Vietnam Veterans Readjustment Survey
OEF	Operation Enduring Freedom
OIF	Operation Iraqi Freedom

OR	Odds ratio
p	Probability
PIT	Point-in-time
PTSD	Post-traumatic stress disorder
SAMHSA	Substance Abuse and Mental Health Services Administration
SSDI	Social Security Disability Insurance
SSI	Social Security Supplementary Income
TANF	Temporary Assistance for Needy Families
TCE	Targeted Capacity Expansion
USICH	United States Interagency Council on Homelessness
VA	Veterans Affairs
VAMC	VA Medical Center
VHA	Veterans Health Administration
VISN	Veterans Integrated Service Networks

EVIDENCE REPORT

INTRODUCTION

BACKGROUND

In 2009, President Obama and Secretary Shinseki committed to ending homelessness among Veterans.[1] In support of that effort, the Federal Strategic Plan to Prevent and End Homelessness 2010 developed by the United States Interagency Council on Homelessness (USICH) has established as one of its goals to prevent and end homelessness among Veterans in five years.[2] An understanding of the epidemiology of homelessness among Veterans and the methodological strengths and weaknesses of this evidence base may inform program-planning efforts and future research needs. Understanding the risk factors for homelessness among Veterans and how these risk factors compare to the general population is important in developing identification and prevention programs for Veterans at risk for homelessness. This report was requested by VA Central Office and The National Center for Homelessness Among Veterans as part of that effort to identify what's known and what's not known about the prevalence of homelessness among Veterans, and about the risk factors for homelessness among Veterans, including risk factors related to military service and incarceration. Given the scope of this assignment and our awareness of other comprehensive review efforts examining the literature on the effectiveness of interventions designed to reduce homelessness, this report focuses on the characteristics, both individual and social, associated with homelessness among Veterans.

Contextual Information: Structural Risk Factors for Homelessness

Any discussion of risk factors for homelessness would be incomplete without acknowledging the complex and multi-dimensional interaction of individual and structural risk factors. Research has consistently demonstrated that structural factors such as lack of affordable housing, cuts in income assistance programs, and labor market changes have created social conditions that have fostered an increase in the homeless population in contemporary U.S. society. For contextual purposes, we include here a brief discussion of this evidence. Much of the literature on structural risk factors focuses on the general homeless population, and is therefore not Veteran specific. However, these structural risk factors for homelessness create a societal context that likely affects Veterans in much the same way as it does the homeless population in general, so a brief background discussion of these issues is relevant.

Lack of Affordable Housing

Lack of affordable housing has been recognized as one of the main structural causes of homelessness in the general population.[3-7] Over the past three decades there has been a dramatic decrease in the availability of affordable housing units for low income renters. In 1970 there was a surplus of 500,000 affordable housing units.[8] By 2008, Extremely Low Income (ELI) renter households, defined as earning less than 30 percent of the median income for the metropolitan area or rural county where they live, experienced a deficit of 3.1 million units.[9] In addition, rental assistance programs such as the Section 8 program, which enables low income households to afford rents in privately owned units, have not been able to assist more than a small number of those who qualify. Only about one-third of those who qualify for housing assistance occupied subsidized housing.[10] It is estimated that the current gap between the number of affordable housing units and the number of people needing them is the largest on record, at 4.4 million units.[9]

Diminishing Employment Prospects

A labor market shift from well paying jobs to minimum wage jobs with fewer benefits has had a direct affect on homelessness. A 2007 survey by the U.S. Conference of Mayors found that 17.4 percent of homeless adults in families were employed, while 13 percent of homeless single adults or unaccompanied youth were employed.[11] For workers earning minimum wage, the real value of their pay has fallen considerably during the past several decades. For instance, the real value of minimum wage fell 26 percent from 1979 to 2004, the last year for which we were able to find such data.[11] The decrease in the real value of income for minimum wage earners has had a significant impact on their ability to pay for housing.[9] Between 1997 and 2005, the number of working families paying more than 50 percent of their income for housing increased 87 percent from 2.4 million to 4.5 million. Among renters alone, the increase in the number of working families who spend more than 50 percent on housing increased 103 percent, from 1 million to 2.1 million.[12] Currently, 71 percent of extremely low income renters spend more than half of their income on rent.[9] Furthermore, unemployment has risen sharply in recent years. At the beginning of the current recession (December 2007), the Bureau of Labor Statistics reported that the number of unemployed persons was 7.7 million, with an unemployment rate of five percent. In July 2010, the number of unemployed persons was 14.7 million with an unemployment rate of 9.5 percent. The number of people experiencing long-term unemployment (27 weeks or longer) grew from 22 percent to 45 percent of the unemployed (from 2.6 million to 6.6 million) between December 2008 and July 2010.[9]

Decrease in Entitlement Payments

A series of policy changes with regard to federal entitlements has steadily eroded the real dollar value of both Supplemental Security Income (SSI) and Aid to Families with Dependent Children (AFCD) payments, now called Temporary Assistance for Needy Families (TANF). The monthly purchasing power of a family receiving AFDC fell by almost one-third, from $568 in 1970 to $385 in 1984. Because of tightened eligibility criteria the number of people who have been able to rely on the government for support has been reduced.[8] The purchasing power of entitlement payments plays a significant role in the ability to secure housing. The fair market rent (FMR) for a two-bedroom unit ($959) exceeds the entire maximum AFDC grant for a mother with two children in every state except Alaska,[13] and is greater than the 2010 maximum federal monthly Social Security Disability Insurance (SSDI) payment of $674.[9] Furthermore, only 10 to 15 percent of homeless individuals received SSI or SSDI assistance, most often because they do not know they qualify or they fail to complete the application process.[14]

METHODS

TOPIC DEVELOPMENT

Key questions for this review were developed with the input of experts from the National Center for Homelessness Among Veterans and the VA New England Healthcare System, and with feedback from national experts on homelessness and homelessness among Veterans (see Appendix B).

The final key questions are:

Key Questions #1a. What is the prevalence and incidence of homelessness among Veterans?

#1b. How has the prevalence and incidence of homelessness among Veterans changed over time?

#1c. How prevalent are psychiatric illness, substance abuse, and chronic medical illness among homeless Veterans?

Key Questions #2a. Which risk factors are associated with new homelessness or a return to homelessness among Veterans? How do these risk factors differ from non-Veteran populations?

#2b. Have risk factors for homelessness among Veterans changed over time?

Key Question #3. Are there factors specific to military service that increase the risk of homelessness, or is the increased risk a marker for pre-military comorbidities and social support deficiencies?

Key Question #4. What is the relationship between incarceration and homelessness among Veterans?

SEARCH STRATEGY

To answer these questions, we began with a horizon scan for any studies or reviews of studies about homelessness and Veterans. The search was performed in December 2009 in MEDLINE (coverage: 1947-present) and the Cochrane Database of Systematic Reviews (coverage: 1993-present), with no limitations on publication year. A supplementary search was conducted in Sociological Abstracts (coverage: 1952-present). Searches in those databases covered the literature available from the beginning of their coverage year through December 2009, and were updated to include coverage through July 2010. We also monitored Table of Contents alerts for several publications to indentify new research published in 2010. To answer Key Question #3, we conducted an additional search of several non-medical qualitative journals, including *Qualitative Research* and *Qualitative Health Research*, with keyword searches on (homeless) AND (military OR combat OR veteran). To answer Key Question #4, we conducted a broad search of MEDLINE, Sociological Abstracts, and Criminal Justice Abstracts (coverage: 1968-present) to identify any studies or reviews of studies of Veterans and incarceration. Keyword searches were conducted in each database for any articles including ((veteran*) AND (jail OR incarcerat* OR prison*)). In addition, a supplementary search of Google Scholar was conducted, looking for any articles meeting the criteria (allintitle: veteran incarcerate OR incarcerated OR incarceration OR prison OR prisoner OR jail). Google Scholar searches were limited to title words because of the large number of articles returned by a more general keyword search.

We sought additional key sources outside indexed journals from homeless researchers and policy-makers identified through snowball sampling (Appendix B). For all key questions, the reference lists of articles returned were reviewed for any additional relevant studies.

STUDY SELECTION

Because of the exploratory nature of this review, few restrictions were placed on articles to be considered for inclusion. Abstracts and full-text articles were not dual reviewed for inclusion. The authors each had responsibility for specific key questions, and reviewed abstracts and full-text articles for those key questions to identify any that might have relevance to the topic of prevalence, risk factors, psychiatric disorders, substance abuse, or chronic medical conditions (VC), military and combat related issues (AT), and incarceration and diversion (HB).

DATA SYNTHESIS

The existing evidence base relevant to this topic does not lend itself to a quantitative synthesis, since sample populations and variables investigated were rarely consistent across studies. In this report, we did not conduct a quantitative data synthesis or meta-analysis, but rather focused on presenting the strength of each existing study's findings and developing a conceptual model for understanding what these findings mean collectively, as well as indicating where there are significant gaps in our knowledge on this topic.

CONCEPTUAL MODEL

Based on a preliminary review of the evidence, the authors developed a conceptual model that provided an analytic framework for understanding the connections between risk factors investigated in different studies. Initially focused on the specific risk factors associated with military service, our conceptual model grew to include pre-military risk factors, as well as factors that, in their general definition, are not unique to Veterans (low or unstable income, for example). We constructed a visual model (Figure 1) to help qualitatively identify the experiences and intermediate outcomes that may be relevant in understanding Veteran homelessness. The conceptual model evolved out of our review and is grounded in the available evidence, with those associations supported by more than one study marked by solid lines, while associations shown by only one study, or where existing evidence is inconsistent, indicated by dashed lines.

A few comments on the assumptions and rationale behind the model are in order. First, several exposures with the same strength of associational evidence are grouped together in one box. This is the case with "low income/low social support/arrests and convictions" and again with all the pre-military service exposures examined. This was done for two reasons: to simplify the model and to graphically suggest that it is likely these exposures interact with one another in ways which are not well isolated or identified in existing research. As is frequently acknowledged in the literature, risk factors for homelessness rarely occur in isolation. Second, the model includes two "black boxes" representing the presence of unmeasured variables. While the primary purpose of the model is to represent what is currently known based on evidence, a secondary purpose of the model is to conceptually make sense of the evidence. Where the mechanism or mediating factors linking two statistically associated variables has not been adequately explored – as, for example, in one study associating Military Sexual Trauma (MST) directly with homelessness – the evidence passes through the black box. In contrast, research investigating low social support, low or unstable income, and arrests/convictions generally makes a clear case for the ways in which these exposures place one at risk for homelessness, and thus no mediating box is included. Third, time is included in the model, which allows the direction of the association to be assumed in some cases (as with early life exposures).

The strength of the associations as indicated in the model is based upon the strength of existing evidence for the Veteran population, but it attempts to indicate how Veteran-specific exposures impact what we have called the "shared exposures," i.e., those common to the general homeless population in the United States. One strength of this model is that it allows the reader to conceptualize the relationships among risk factors unique to the experience of Veterans together with risk factors common to broader populations of homeless individuals. For example, the association between low social support and homelessness is a general one that has been observed in other homeless populations, as has the association between low social support and mental illness. However, the association between mental illness and combat exposure is unique to Veterans. We feel it may be important for future intervention efforts to understand these Veteran-unique exposures and their impact on shared exposures, and have thus highlighted them in this report, even as we conclude that homeless Veterans have much in common with the non-Veteran homeless.

This conceptual model, though derived independently by the review team and more inclusive of structural risk factors, bears similarities to the model put forward by Rosenheck and Fontana (1994), who looked at data from the National Vietnam Veterans Readjustment Survey (NVVRS) to investigate risk factors for Veteran homelessness.[15] The NVVRS was a landmark attempt to understand the impact of the Vietnam War on both the physical and social health of Veterans, and no study to date has replicated its nationally representative, mixed-methods data collection design for investigating multiple risk factors. The current generation of Veterans who have experienced the conflicts in Iraq and Afghanistan may exhibit different characteristics and is deserving of research of similar scope.

PEER REVIEW

A draft version of this report was reviewed by six experts in the field of homelessness. Their comments and our responses are presented in Appendix A.

A Critical Review of the Literature Regarding Homelessness among Veterans

Figure 1. Risk Factors for Veteran Homelessness: Conceptual Model

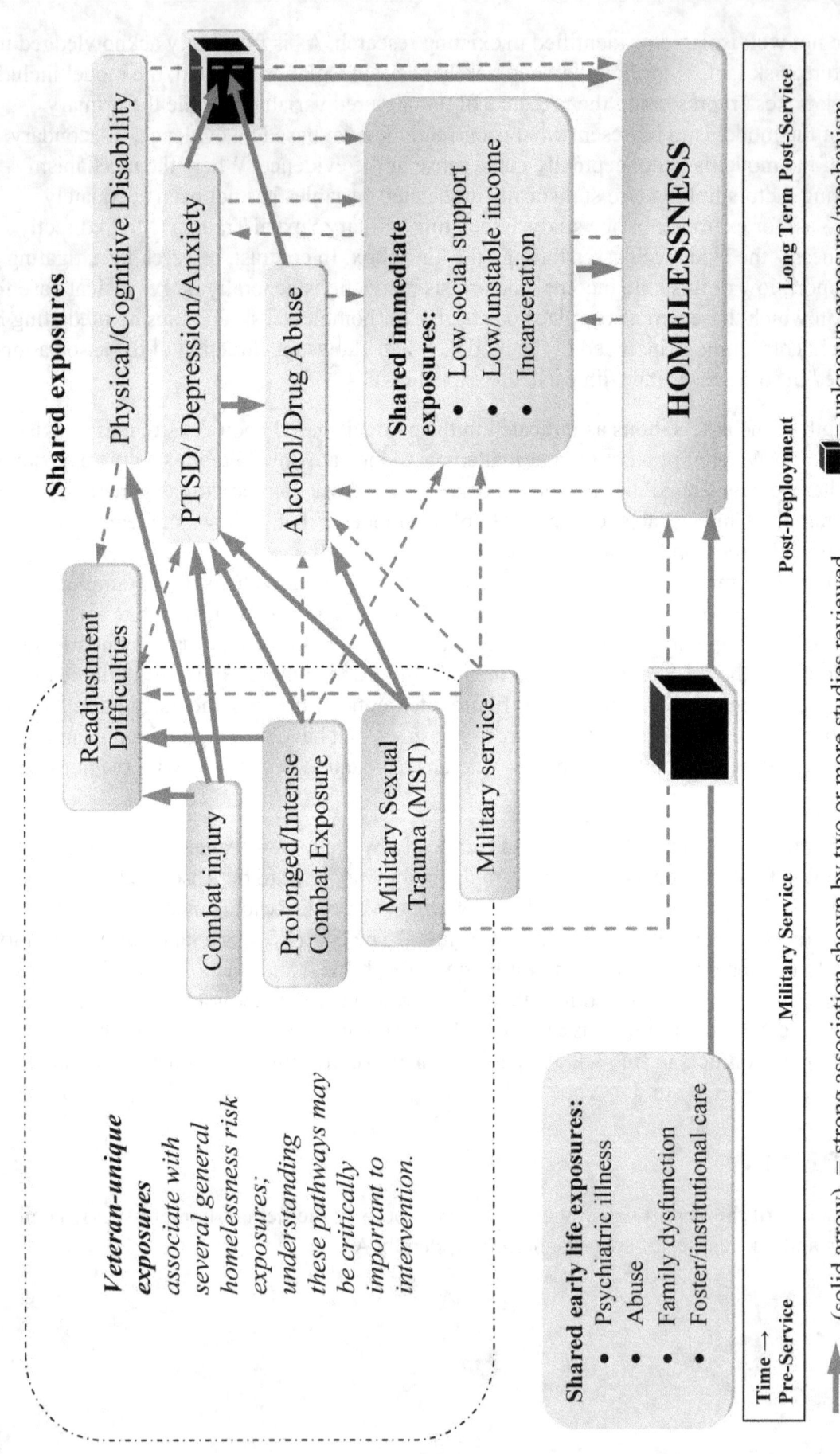

RESULTS

DEFINITIONS OF HOMELESSNESS

The current definition of a "homeless Veteran" combines both Veteran status and homeless status. The VA considers a Veteran as a person who "served in the active military, naval, or air service" and was not dishonorably discharged. However, many studies of homeless Veterans include as a Veteran anyone who reports having served in the military, regardless of active duty or discharge status. Reported Veteran status is rarely confirmed through a review of VA administrative data. Veterans are considered homeless if they meet the definition of "homeless individual" established by the McKinney-Vento Homeless Act (P.L. 100-77). The McKinney-Vento Act defines a homeless individual as an individual who lacks a fixed, regular, and adequate nighttime residence, and a person who had a nighttime residence that is: a supervised publically or privately operated shelter designed to provide temporary living accommodations; an institution that provides a temporary residence for individuals intended to be institutionalized; or a public or private place not designed for or ordinarily used as a regular sleeping accommodation for human beings.[16]

The current definition of homelessness under the McKinney-Vento Act does not include those living in transitional housing not exclusively for the mentally ill, those who are in imminent threat of losing their housing, those fleeing a situation of domestic violence or other life-threatening condition, as well as unaccompanied youth and certain types of homeless families with children. Recent amendments to McKinney-Vento through the Homeless Emergency and Rapid Transition to Housing (HEARTH) Act will expand the definition of homelessness to include these families and individuals.[16] Changes in the definition of who is counted as homeless were scheduled to go into effect in November, 2010. These changes, along with demographic changes in the nature of the military, particularly among those serving in the Operation Iraqi Freedom (OIF) and Operation Enduring Freedom (OEF) era, and as a result of the increase in women serving in the military, are likely to have an impact both on the numbers and needs of homeless Veterans and their families.[16]

ASSESSING THE LIMITATIONS OF THE CURRENT RESEARCH

There are several limitations of the studies that have examined the individual level risk factors for homelessness.

Problems in Sampling and Populations

Sampling limitations are common. Most studies include samples that disproportionately comprise the chronically homeless rather than the newly homeless. Studies often rely on small, geographically isolated samples, which make it difficult to make generalizations about the larger homeless population.[17-19] In addition, several studies examine former homeless individuals, often termed "ever homeless," in order to draw more generalizable conclusions about the homeless experience. Although such studies are useful, their sample selection includes only those, who for whatever reason, have made it out of homelessness, thus undersampling those who may have higher rates of symptom severity for risk factors such as substance abuse and mental illness.

Few studies directly assess the prevalence of psychiatric, substance abuse, or chronic illness in the general population of homeless Veterans. Most studies rely on already morbid populations seeking treatment for services and so cannot provide estimates of prevalence in the population as a whole. Fischer and Breakey[20] further point out that much research has relied on nonrandom sampling frames, which may introduce bias, thus influencing prevalence rates of certain attributes. Rates of alcohol, drug, and mental health problems, for instance, tend to appear larger among homeless individuals sampled in shelters, clinics and on the streets; and lower in sampling sites such as food or service providers.[20]

Comparators

Few studies include appropriate housed control groups to determine the difference in prevalence for certain risk factors. Matched for race, gender, and age, census data or large household surveys give a sense of the differences in the homeless population as compared to the general housed population, but a more narrowly focused control group of marginally housed individuals living in poverty would present a more accurate picture of the predictive factors that are related to homelessness. Studies that include univariate comparisons often do so without calculating risk ratios.[19-22]

Settings

Research on homelessness is often conducted in service settings, including shelters and rehabilitation centers, which increases the chance of over-representing the chronically homeless and under-representing those who are homeless for short periods of time. Because the chronic homeless tend to have higher rates of substance abuse and mental illness, an over-representation of the chronically homeless will result in an overestimation of such characteristics.[23] Thus, choice of sampling site affects prevalence rates.[21]

Definitions

Existing studies also frequently differ in the definitions of key dependent variables, including homelessness itself. Some studies interpret homelessness as literal homelessness (sleeping in a shelter or on the street), while other studies include more liberal definitions. Some studies examine the dichotomy of ever/never being homeless, while others employ a strict point-in-time or cross-sectional definition and do not collect data on sample participants' lifetime experience of homelessness.

Measures and Measurement Issues

Measurements used to operationalize the included risk factors have not been consistent. For example, social support in some cases is measured as "having someone close to you that can provide support," while other studies use marital status as a surrogate to determine the level of one's social support status. Even questions regarding Veteran status can lead to different estimates. Asking, "Are you a Veteran?" for example, can generate a different response than asking, "Did you serve in the armed forces?" In addition, studies do not always include the same variables in their models. Several studies failed to include variables that have been found significant in other research, such as childhood adversity, employment history and former incarceration, and so may not adequately control for possible confounders. In addition, structural factors such as housing affordability or job market conditions have largely been left out of the research design in many of the studies examining risk factors for homelessness, although they have largely been significant in the models that have included them.[22] Thus, it is impossible to determine if controlling for structural risk factors would have altered the results of such research.

In addition to the methodological inconsistencies described above, we found great variability in the methods and instruments used to determine the prevalence of alcohol abuse, substance abuse, and mental illness among homeless Veterans. The type of measurement used (current use, past use, or lifetime use) is also largely inconsistent. We found that a large percentage of studies have based their findings on self-report (which depends greatly on the willingness of self-disclosure of study participants) or on instruments in which there is no clear evidence of validation for the homeless population. Differences in prevalence between studies using self-report vs. standard instruments can be stark. Fischer and Breakey point out, moreover, that estimates based on prior treatment history may not be accurate because of the various ways in which individuals seek help from service providers. Some patients, for example, seek help through outpatient services and, so, would not be included in counts of hospitalized patients – a common measurement threshold for prevalence estimates of mental illness and substance abuse.[20]

Much of the research that examines the associations between substance abuse/mental illness and homelessness does so from a pathology perspective rather than from an adaptation perspective.[24] By using instruments that are designed primarily for use on clinical populations, such research may misinterpret adaptive behaviors as pathology. We suggest that researchers should provide evidence of validation for the instruments used when reporting the associations between substance abuse and/or mental illness among homeless Veterans. By addressing the validation of instruments used on the homeless population, researchers will be able to draw a more accurate picture of the risk factors associated with homelessness among Veterans.

Study Design

Many of the studies examining Veteran homelessness employ a cross-sectional research design, which limits the interpretation of cause and effect regarding substance abuse/mental illness and homelessness. Thus, in many cases, it is unclear as to whether substance abuse and/or mental illness preceded homelessness, or if substance abuse and/or mental illness are the result of adaptations to the stresses and dangers associated with the homeless experience.

Summary of Limitations

Because of the inconsistencies in the instruments used and the inherent differences found in study design, comparisons across studies are problematic. We agree with Fischer and Breakey that comparisons of studies should take into account differences in problem definition, method of assessment, sampling techniques, and demographic characteristics of the sample.[20]

DATA SOURCES

A recent Government Accounting Office (GAO) review of Federal data and other studies on homelessness concluded that "these data have a number of shortcomings and consequently do not capture the true extent and nature of homelessness."[25] While that review was broadly focused on data on homeless populations in general, it did include a review of data available on homeless Veterans, and many of its findings are equally applicable to data on the Veteran sub-population.

Annual Homeless Assessment Report (AHAR) and Community Homelessness Assessment, Local Education, and Networking Group (CHALENG) Report Data

There are three current data sources widely relied on for estimating the number of homeless Veterans:

- The AHAR provides estimates of Veteran homelessness from two data sources:
  - the Department of Housing and Urban Development's (HUD's) Point-in-Time (PIT) estimate, that gives an approximation of the number of homeless individuals and families during a single night in January;
  - the Homeless Management Information System (HMIS) estimates, which produce counts of the sheltered homeless population during a calendar year; and
- The annual CHALENG for Veterans report uses a combination of data sources to determine a count of Veteran homelessness.

PIT estimates are gathered on a single night during the last week in January. Continuum of Care (CoC) applications are submitted to HUD annually as part of the competitive funding process and provide one-night, PIT estimates of both sheltered and unsheltered homeless populations.[14] Information about homeless subgroups are also collected.

HMIS are electronic administrative databases that are designed to record and store client-level information on the characteristics and service needs of homeless persons. HMIS data are used to produce counts of the sheltered homeless population over a full year. It includes people who used emergency shelter or transitional housing programs at some time during the course of a year.[14]

Since 1994, the VA has estimated the number of Veterans receiving services in its CHALENG program. Estimates are derived through partnerships with representatives from each local VA medical center (VAMC) and service providers from state and local governments and nonprofit organizations. Using a point-in-time estimate, each VAMC estimates the greatest number of Veterans who are homeless on any given day in the previous fiscal year. Various sources are used to arrive at the estimates and include HUD PIT counts, previous Census estimates, VA client data, VA staff impressions, or combinations of sources.[26]

Estimates from the most recent CHALENG report are based on PIT estimates of the number of Veterans homeless on any day during the last week of January 2008. While these estimates include both sheltered and unsheltered Veterans, like all PIT estimates, the CHALENG count is likely to undercount those who are not chronically homeless. In addition, these estimates are often adjusted to better align with estimates based on the HUD PIT count, noting that "CHALENG has increasingly relied upon HUD PIT counts as the basis of its own estimate."[26] The reasons for this are unclear. This approach establishes the HUD count as a gold standard despite the CHALENG authors' own acknowledgment that the HUD PIT counts may not have included areas with concentrations of homeless Veterans known by those responsible for the CHALENG estimate.[26]

HUD and the VA have recently collaborated in producing and releasing a Veteran-specific supplement to the annual AHAR. This report *Veteran Homelessness: A Supplemental Report to the 2009 Annual Homeless Assessment Report to Congress*[27] (2009 Veteran AHAR) is a major contribution to our understanding of the extent and nature of homelessness among Veterans. The report is based on PIT and HMIS data collected as described above using a standard, validated method to minimize potential duplication in the count, and with statistical adjustments made to account for undercounting. The 2009 Veteran AHAR provides national one-day and one-year estimates of homeless Veterans and describes their demographic characteristics and patterns of shelter use. We recommend that the Veteran AHAR be used as the most comprehensive and reliable source of information on the prevalence of homelessness among Veterans currently available. The report is available at: http://www.hudhre.info/documents/2009AHARVeteransReport.pdf.

Our report should be seen as a complementary report that provides a critical review of the research and literature on homelessness among Veterans.

In addition to the AHAR and CHALENG counts, which attempt to provide national estimates of the number of homeless Veterans, other data sources are used to provide estimates of subpopulations of homeless Veterans and their individual characteristics, and to identify risk factors for homelessness among Veterans. What follows is an overview of some of the more central of those data sources. This is not intended to be a comprehensive review of all data sources on homeless Veterans; rather, it is a review of what we consider to have been a core set of those data sources – those that have been consistently used in a number of studies, and those which we consider exemplars of the strengths and weaknesses of data on homeless Veterans.

National Vietnam Veterans Readjustment Study (NVVRS)

One of the earliest sources of data on Veteran homelessness and on related factors such as drug and alcohol use and post-traumatic stress disorder (PTSD) was the NVVRS. Conducted between September 1984 and November 1988, this study of 1,200 Veterans provided a representative sample of all persons on active duty in the U.S. military during the Vietnam War era (August 5, 1964 through May 7, 1975).

Although it was a well-conducted study, the population may not be representative of post-Vietnam era Veterans. Theater Veterans of the Vietnam War era were younger and less likely to be female or minorities than subsequent Veteran cohorts. They also served during a period of a military draft – while Veterans of the post-Vietnam era served in an all volunteer military, over 40 percent of the respondents to the NVVRS had been drafted or enlisted to avoid the draft. While in 1974, 60 percent of the active duty force were age 25 or younger, by 2000, that percentage had declined to 46 percent; and while in 1974, only 3 percent of the active duty force were women and 20 percent were minorities, by 2000, women accounted for 15 percent and minorities 35 percent of those on active duty.[28] Since the Vietnam era, the military has also seen an increase in service members with family obligations.[29]

Two current studies, the Health of Vietnam Era Veteran Women's Study (Health VIEWS)[30] and the Millennium Cohort Study (MCS),[31] may provide additional information on the prevalence of risk factors for homelessness among women Veterans (Health VIEWS) and among OEF-OIF Veterans (MCS).

National Survey of Homeless Assistance Providers and Clients (NSHAPC)

One of the most widely used sources of information on homelessness in general, as well as on homelessness among Veterans, is the NSHAPC. This survey was conducted between October 18, 1996 and November 14, 1996 and included a nationally representative sample of over 4,000 homeless clients of nearly 12,000 homeless assistance providers. The survey collected data on, among other things, Veteran status, mental health, drug and alcohol use, and homelessness status (currently or formerly). While in 1996, 13 percent of adult U.S. population were Veterans, 23 percent of the then currently homeless clients were Veterans. Considering males only, 33 percent of the male homeless clients were Veterans compared with 31 percent of the adult male U.S. population.

While a number of later studies of homelessness among Veterans made use of the NSHAPC data, several limitations to the data should be noted. First, the study includes information only on clients of services for the homeless and does not include information on the homeless who did not access services. It also entirely excludes the homeless in communities that had few or no homeless assistance programs. In addition, all client data, including data on physical and mental health problems, use of alcohol and drugs, and incarceration were based on self-report. Finally, because the survey collected data on homelessness was only for the period of one month, as with all point-in-time surveys, it will likely reflect a bias towards those who are chronically as opposed to episodically or temporarily homeless.

Health Care for Homeless Veterans (HCHV)

Many of the studies of homelessness among Veterans are based on data from clinical populations receiving services in VA programs, and so may have limited applicability to an understanding of homelessness among Veterans more generally. While these are often large national data sets, they nevertheless capture data only on those Veterans participating in those programs. In addition, these programs are often focused on Veterans with particularly acute service needs. A description of some of the programs most frequently used as sources of data follows.

Homeless Chronically Mentally Ill Veterans Program (HCMI)

The HCMI program was established in 1987 at 43 Veteran Administration Medical Centers in 26 states and the District of Columbia as a program for Veterans with psychiatric problems. An initial assessment of the program conducted between May 1987 and March 1988 found that the median age of participants was 40 (younger than Veterans in the general population); that 67 percent needed specialized psychiatric, and 72 percent needed medical evaluation or treatment: that 46 percent reported significant substance abuse and 65 percent reported a previous hospitalization for either a psychiatric or substance abuse problem; that 47 percent were living in shelters, 9 percent were doubling up, 8 percent had a room or apartment, and 35 percent had no residence; and that over half were Vietnam era Veterans.

Domiciliary Care for Homeless Veterans (DCHV)

The DCHV program was also established in 1987 as a 20-site expansion of the VA's existing domiciliary care program. It was targeted at Veterans who were either medically or psychiatrically disabled, and who were either homeless or at imminent risk for homelessness. In an initial assessment of the program conducted between November 1987 and November 1988, nearly 90 percent of admitted Veterans received major psychiatric or substance abuse diagnoses; 69 percent had been hospitalized at a VAMC for a substance abuse, psychiatric, or medical problem in the previous year; 47 percent had a current substance abuse problem, 36 percent a current psychiatric problem, and 16 percent were dual diagnosed; and 54 percent had a serious chronic, medical illness.

Access to Community Care and Effective Service Supports (ACCESS)

The ACCESS program was established by Substance Abuse and Mental Health Services Administration (SAMHSA) in 1993 as a five-year demonstration project to identify effective approaches to providing services to homeless persons with serious mental illnesses. Clients were eligible for case management services if they were homeless, suffered from severe mental illness, and were not involved in ongoing treatment in the community. Of those who eventually enrolled in the case management phase of the program, 67 percent were diagnosed with a psychotic disorder (37 percent with schizophrenia, 32 percent with other psychoses, 20 percent with bipolar disorder), 49 percent were diagnosed with major depression, 22 percent with personality disorder, and/or 19 percent with anxiety disorder (diagnoses are not mutually exclusive); 43 percent were diagnosed with alcohol abuse; and 38 percent were diagnosed with drug abuse.

METHODOLOGICAL CONSIDERATIONS

Estimates of the number of homeless are sensitive both to the definitions of homelessness (who is deemed homeless) and the methods for counting the homeless population.[21, 23] Point-in-time estimates are more likely to capture the chronically homeless population than HMIS counts, and may undercount those who are transitionally or episodically homeless. The HMIS counts, however, are sensitive to under-reporting, since CoCs are not required to submit HMIS data. The Veteran AHAR statistically adjusts the raw count to account for undercounting in the PIT estimate of one-day sheltered and unsheltered homelessness, and uses statistical adjustments and weighting of the HMIS to produce national one-year estimates of the sheltered homeless.[27] The accuracy of those estimates will be sensitive to the validity of the assumptions underlying the adjustments. Appendix A of the Veteran AHAR provides a description of the methodology used to adjust the PIT counts,[27] and Appendix B.5 of the 2009 AHAR provides a description of the methods used to adjust and weight the HMIS estimate.[14]

There are several data collection issues that make estimating the number of homeless Veterans difficult. Those who are doubled up with family or friends but who would otherwise be without shelter are generally not included in homeless samples.[32] Estimates of Veteran homelessness often will miss the hidden homeless who sleep in automobiles, in campgrounds or in other areas not easily identified by researchers, as well as those who may intentionally hide from researchers.[32]

KEY QUESTION #1A. What is the prevalence and incidence of homelessness among Veterans?

For reasons discussed earlier in the Limitations section, the exact number of homeless Veterans is unknown. The most recent CHALENG for Veterans report estimates that on on a single night in January 2008 there were 107,000 homeless Veterans.[26] This represents a decrease of 18 percent from the estimate of 131,000 homeless Veterans reported in the 2008 CHALENG report.[26] It is argued that this is primarily the result of changes in counting methods rather than an actual decline in the number of homeless Veterans.[33] The CHALENG report further speculates that improved methods (such as adjusting estimates to better coincide with local HUD PIT counts), VA program interventions, changing demographics, and recent events (i.e., reduction in estimates due to ongoing recovery from the effects of Hurricane Katrina) may have had an impact on the reported prevalence of homelessness among Veterans.[26] With nearly 23 million Veterans in the U.S. population in 2008, and an estimated 107,000 homeless, the rate of homelessness among Veterans was approximately 47 for every 10,000 Veterans. This rate is more than double the rate of homelessness in the general adult population.[14]

The recently released 2009 Veteran AHAR estimates that on a single night in January 2009 there were 75,609 homeless Veterans and that an estimated 136,334 Veterans spent at least one night in an emergency shelter or transitional housing program between October 1, 2008 and September 30, 2009.[27] Based on the Veteran AHAR estimate of 75,609 homeless Veterans on a single night in January 2009, approximately 33 of every 10,000 Veterans were homeless.

In 2009, Veterans made up just under 10 percent of the U.S. adult population, and over 11 percent of the adults in emergency shelters or transitional housing between October 1, 2008 and September 30, 2009. This accounts for 1 of every 168 Veterans in the U.S. or 1 in every 10 Veterans living in poverty.[27] In addition, it has been argued that from 89,553 to 467,877 Veterans are at risk for homelessness.[33] In the United States, men in general are more likely to be homeless than women, and the Veteran population continues to be disproportionately male, so some of this increased risk can be ascribed to this. However, while females comprise only 6.8 percent of the total Veteran population, they made up 7.5 percent of homeless Veterans.[27]

While Blacks make up only 11 percent of the overall Veteran population, they were 34 percent of the homeless Veterans. Similarly, Hispanics comprise only 5 percent of all Veterans, but 11 percent of homeless Veterans; and American Indian and Alaska Natives, while comprising less 1 percent of all Veterans, were over 3 percent of the homeless Veterans.[27]

In 2009, nearly half of all Veterans were between the ages of 31 and 50, and over a third were between 51 and 61. Over 11,000 Veterans between the ages of 18 and 30 used an emergency shelter or transitional housing in 2009, suggesting a potential growing need to address the problem of homelessness among Veterans of Operation Iraqi Freedom and Operation Enduring Freedom.[27]

KEY QUESTION #1B. How has the prevalence and incidence of homelessness among Veterans changed over time?

Because of changes in reporting and in the methods for counting the number of homeless, estimates of the prevalence of homelessness among Veterans over time are not comparable. The 16th CHALENG report estimated that there were 107,000 Veterans homeless on a single day in January 2008.[26] In contrast, the 2009 Veteran AHAR estimates that there were 75,609 homeless Veterans on a single night in January 2009.[27] While this 30 percent decrease in the number of homeless could be real, it is more likely an artifact of changes in the methods for counting and adjusting estimates; therefore, we suggest caution when using previous estimates to examine changes in prevalence over time. HUD and the VA intend to continue to collaborate on future annual Veteran supplements to the AHAR which should result in more consistent estimates for tracking trends in homelessness among Veterans.

However, even these new estimates should be interpreted with caution for several reasons. First, as HUD points out, the HMIS data on Veteran status are for sheltered homeless only. Some researchers have speculated that Veterans, are more likely than other homeless groups to remain unsheltered.[14] Second, some of the residential programs for the homeless that are funded through the U.S. Department of Veterans Affairs do not report data to the CoC. Moreover, there is anecdotal evidence that homeless Veterans do not always reveal their Veteran status to program staff.[14]

It has been speculated that the number of homeless Veterans will increase, as Veterans return from OEF and OIF suffer from high rates of mental illness and traumatic brain injury; these and other returning Veterans may experience problems in obtaining employment within the civil sector.[34] The accuracy of these speculations may not be known for many years, as historically Veteran homelessness usually occurs long after return to civilian life. In a study of over 1,400 homeless males, 76 percent of combat Veterans and half of all noncombat Veterans first became homeless more than a decade after leaving military service.[35] In addition, the demographic composition of the Veteran homeless population is changing. As documented by Kuhn et al. (2010), VA facilities recently reported an increase of 24 percent in homeless Veteran families seeking services from those facilities. Indeed, family issues such as child care were among the top 10 needs reported by homeless individuals in the most recent CHALENG survey.[26] A recent study assessing risk factors for homelessness among female Veterans found that 16 percent of homeless Veterans had children under the age of 18 living with them during the prior 12 months.[36] The percentage of homeless women Veterans is expected to increase as the percentage of female Veterans has increased dramatically in recent years. Over 165,000 female troops have been deployed to Iraq and Afghanistan, a much higher number than deployed during the Vietnam and Gulf Wars.[16] Researchers should remain alert to the possibility that changing demographics within the military may, in the future, be associated with different, potentially more rapid paths to homelessness.

KEY QUESTION #1C. How prevalent are psychiatric illness, substance abuse, and chronic medical illness among homeless Veterans?

There are few studies directly assessing the prevalence of psychiatric, substance abuse, or chronic illness in the general population of homeless Veterans. Most studies rely on already morbid populations seeking treatment for services and so cannot provide estimates of prevalence in the population as a whole. Of the studies we located which focus on substance abuse and mental illness among homeless Veterans, we found very little consistency in the methods and instruments used to determine the prevalence of substance abuse and mental illness. The type of measurement (current use, past use, and lifetime use) was also inconsistent, which can greatly affect reported prevalence rates, as those reporting lifetime drug abuse or mental illness will have higher rates compared with those reporting current abuse or illness. It is also difficult to determine from the included studies if distinctions were made between hazardous use, abuse, and dependence. The severity of abuse has implications for functioning, risk, and capacity to engage in services.

Several studies have based their findings on self-report, a method which depends greatly on the willingness and accuracy of self-disclosure of study participants, or on instruments for which it is unclear if they have been validated with homeless populations. Differences in prevalence between studies using self-report vs. those using standard instruments can be substantial. Fischer and Breakey[20] point out, moreover, that estimates based on prior treatment history may not be accurate because of the various ways in which individuals seek help from service providers. Some patients, for example, seek help through outpatient services and thus would not be included in counts of hospitalized patients – a common measurement threshold for prevalence estimates of mental illness and substance abuse. Because of these inconsistencies, comparisons across studies are problematic.

Furthermore, many of the studies examining Veteran homelessness employed a cross-sectional research design, which limits the interpretation of cause and effect regarding substance abuse/mental illness and homelessness. Nevertheless, we feel that the evidence is adequate and consistent enough with evidence regarding the prevalence of these conditions in homeless populations in general,[21, 22, 37] to state that the prevalence of mental health, substance abuse, and medical problems among Veteran homeless is high, despite access to Veteran Health Administration (VHA) services.

Existing evidence suggests that homeless Veterans have higher rates of substance abuse (drug and alcohol abuse), mental illness, and chronic illness when compared to housed Veterans. However, here, too, estimates vary. A study based on a convenience sample of homeless adults admitted to homeless shelters in Santa Clara County, California between November 1989 and March 1990 found that 17 percent of Veterans had been admitted for overnight treatment of psychiatric problems, 29 percent reported actual and 39 percent perceived alcohol abuse, and 22 percent reported illegal drug use.[35] More recently, in a cross-sectional, community-based survey of homeless male Veterans (N=127) and non-Veterans (N=298) in Pittsburgh and Philadelphia during a five-month period in 1997, O'Toole et al.[37] sampled from emergency shelters, transitional and supportive housing units, and soup kitchens or drop-in sites to ensure adequate representation of all homeless persons. That study found that 61.4 percent of homeless Veterans reported psychiatric problems, 79.5 percent reported alcohol or drug abuse or dependence, and 66.1 percent reported having at least one chronic medical condition.[37] In addition, Veterans were more likely to report a chronic medical condition than non-Veterans (66% vs. 55%, p = 0.04). Of the 127 male Veterans included in the study, 24 percent reported hypertension, 19 percent hepatitis/cirrhosis, and 7 percent each diabetes and heart disease, while 36 percent reported two or more chronic conditions. Of note, the usual sources of care for the Veteran population were shelter-based clinics (48 percent) as opposed to community clinics (35 percent). As a whole, homeless Veterans have higher rates of chronic illness compared to homeless non-Veterans, but tend to have similar rates of substance abuse (alcohol or drug abuse) and mental illness when compared to their non-Veteran counterparts, although Veterans tend to have better access to care.[37]

A study of homeless Veterans with physical, mental, and substance abuse disorders seeking treatment from the DCHV Program examined indicators for chronic homelessness. The study consisted of two samples, with both samples including short-term (<12 months since age 18) and chronic (>12 months since age 18) homeless Veterans. The study found chronic homelessness to be associated with substance abuse disorders for both samples, but only one sample showed an association between mental illness (depression and anxiety) and chronic homelessness.[38]

In a secondary analysis of national VAMCs' administrative data on over 40,000 housed and homeless patients receiving inpatient care between 1996 and 1998, Adams et al.[39] found that a significantly greater proportion of homeless patients than housed had a psychiatric disorder (42.1% vs. 22.1%, $p \leq 0.001$) or substance abuse (37.7% vs. 6.9%, $p \leq 0.001$) as a discharge diagnosis. Homeless persons in this study included both the literal homeless and those doubled up, i.e. staying temporarily with family or friends. No major differences were found between housed and homeless Veterans regarding surgical or medical conditions.

KEY QUESTION #2A. Which risk factors are associated with new homelessness or a return to homelessness among Veterans? How do these risk factors differ from non-Veteran populations?

Risk factors most strongly and consistently associated with homelessness include childhood risk factors such as inadequate care by the parents, experiencing foster care or group placement, and prolonged periods of running away from home. These risk factors have also been consistently found to be associated with homelessness in the general population.[21, 40, 41] Overall, homeless Veterans and non-Veterans tend to have similar rates of alcohol and substance abuse.[35, 37] Comparisons of rates of mental illness and overall health status between Veterans and non-Veterans have not found a consistent association across studies.[35, 42]

There do not appear to be differences between Veterans and non-Veterans with regard to some of the factors most immediately associated with homelessness. However, there do appear to be unique, military-related pathways by which Veterans are exposed to these factors, since Veteran-specific exposures such as combat injury, intense or prolonged combat, and Military Sexual Trauma all have an impact on shared exposures such as mental illness and low or unstable income.

There are notable differences in the prevalence of some characteristics often found to be protective. Veteran homeless tend to be older and better educated, have had better early family cohesion, and are more likely to be or have been married than non-Veteran homeless. The reasons for the absence of expected protections are not well understood. It may be that the differences between these populations are too small to influence outcomes significantly. Alternatively, there may be unique Veteran experiences associated with either service or post-deployment readjustment that actively undermine the protective mechanism associated with these factors in other populations. For example, it may be that individuals with strong positive family experiences or high social support in the form of marriage may actually be more negatively affected by the physical and emotional dislocation of combat service than those who have weaker social support networks. Similar arguments have been offered to explain why National Guard Veterans, who are often older, more established in their civilian lives, and less connected to the social supports and services offered to active military post-deployment, are often considered, at least anecdotally, to have particularly severe post-deployment readjustment difficulties.[43] Research is needed to move these explanations beyond mere conjecture, however.

KEY QUESTION #2B. Have risk factors for homelessness among Veterans changed over time?

We found no evidence to suggest that risk factors themselves change over time. What the evidence does show is that over time, certain risk factors become more salient than others and that they affect different sub-populations. Military-related trauma, for instance, has always been a risk factor for the subsequent development of mental illness putting one at risk for homelessness. Historically, the trauma most closely associated with military service has been PTSD, but with the increasing number of women in the military, military sexual trauma (MST) has become an important and prevalent additional trauma-associated risk factor. Similar comments can be made regarding the increasing number of family-involved Veterans. The wars in Iraq and Afghanistan have led to an increase in the number of National Guard Veterans serving often repeated tours of duty in these conflicts. Since these Veterans are more likely to have families during and immediately after deployment, the importance of factors related to homelessness among families has increased. Similarly, if certain aspects of combat experience put Veterans at increased for homelessness – something which the evidence suggests – these will only be relevant risk factors during periods when U.S. forces are engaged in combat missions. Finally, economic and structural factors will strongly influence who is at risk. In good economic times, those most vulnerable because of personal risk factors will become homeless; as economic conditions worsen, an increasing number of those less vulnerable will also become homeless.

KEY QUESTION #3. Are there factors specific to military service that increase the risk of homelessness, or is the increased risk a marker for pre-military comorbidities and social support deficiencies?

Very little research designed to investigate military specific risk factors for homelessness has been conducted. Pre-military risk factors or comorbidities do not account for the over-representation of Veterans among the nation's homeless. Prolonged or intense combat exposure appears to indirectly increase the risk of homelessness through its impact on mental health, employment, and social support.[15, 44-51] Some exposures that may increase the risk of homelessness, like alcohol/drug abuse and low social support, frequently emerge during service or the post-deployment period.[52, 53] Though only examined to date by one small study, MST has been associated with increased risk of homelessness among female Veterans.[36]

No study has comprehensively looked at risk factors for emerging OEF/OIF cohorts of Veterans.

Future research should employ longitudinal study designs and more detailed data concerning combat exposures to track the general population of Veterans' exposures to clearly-defined potential risk factors during active duty and the readjustment/post-deployment period.

Pre-military Risk Factors or Comorbidities Do Not Account for the Over-representation of Veterans among the Nation's Homeless

Some studies have found that homeless Veterans have lower prevalence of some general population risk factors (such as family dysfunction) and higher prevalence of protective factors (such as higher educational levels) when compared with other homeless individuals.[36, 54, 55] These findings suggest that pre-military risk factors or comorbidities do not account for the over-representation of Veterans among the nation's homeless. As has been found for the general population, some childhood risk factors are strongly associated with Veteran homelessness,[15] but the limited evidence available suggests that these risk factors are no more prevalent among Veterans than among the general population. Veterans as a group appear to actually be at decreased risk for some exposures associated with homelessness in the general population.

In bivariate analysis, Rosenheck and Fontana (1994)[15] found an increased risk ratio for homelessness for those who had been in foster care, but only 0.7 percent of their sample had experienced such care. Their structural equation model also found that childhood abuse, childhood trauma and psychiatric treatment before age 18 were all significantly associated with homelessness, but they did not report how the prevalence of these exposures compared with prevalence in the general homeless population.[15] Tessler, Rosenheck and Gamache[55] found that while pre-military misconduct and childhood family instability were both significantly more prevalent among younger cohorts of homeless Veterans compared to older cohorts, overall, Veterans were significantly less likely than the general homeless sample to have experienced either exposure.

In terms of protective factors, Tessler, Rosenheck and Gamache found that homeless Veterans were likely to be slightly (on average < 1 year) more educated than homeless non-Veterans,[55] a finding similar to that of Rosenheck and Koegel's earlier study.[42] This is consistent with the finding that education may be protective against homelessness within Veteran populations, as was found by Washington, Yano and McGuire's[36] small single-site study comparing currently housed and non-housed female Veterans.

Studies examining whether Veterans as a group possess better social support than the general population have produced mixed results, which is likely due, in part, to poor consensus on how to define and measure social support. Marital status is the most common measure of social support, and findings with regard to marriage suggest that homeless Veterans are more likely than homeless non-Veterans to have ever been married.[42, 55] More centrally, the validity of marriage as a useful measure of social support has been questioned; more nuanced and better validated measures such as the Medical Outcomes Study (MOS) Social Support Survey[56] or Lin's Strong Ties Measure[57] would strengthen any findings regarding this risk factor. The NVVRS employed a richer definition of social support, but its findings did not report differences in pre-military social support between overall Veteran and comparison general population.

Rosenheck and Koegel[42] used data from three surveys of homeless service users in 1986-1987 to investigate differences between Veteran and non-Veteran homeless men, and found no significant differences in risk factors associated with physical or psychiatric illness; homeless Veterans were more likely to have been treated in the past for alcohol problems, but the authors suggest that this is likely an artifact of greater access to care through VA services. Though these findings are now dated and ideally should be tested against findings from a more current sample, there is to date no study to contradict Rosenheck and Koegel's conclusion that "veterans appear to be at risk for homelessness for much the same reasons as other American men."[42]

While Veterans thus appear to be at risk for homelessness for much the same structural reasons as other Americans, there are qualitative differences in their pathways of exposure which warrant further research. The influence of unique exposures (such as combat exposure or MST) on more proximate, shared exposures (such as poor mental health) requires research designed specifically to investigate this topic further.

Prolonged or Intense Combat Exposure Indirectly but Substantially Increases the Risk of Homelessness

Two studies that investigated homelessness outcomes in relation to exposures to hypothesized military service risk factors were identified: Rosenheck and Fontana[15] and Washington, Yano and Macguire.[36] Rosenheck and Fontana looked at pre-service, military service (combat exposure and participation in atrocities), and post-service experiences as risk factors for Veterans serving during the Vietnam War era; Washington and colleagues examined military and other sexual trauma among female Veterans of several eras. Rosenheck and Fontana's data allowed for a division of the sample into ever-homeless and never-homeless, while Washington and colleagues did not collect data on past housing status and, in fact, noted in their results that much of their housed population might be at risk for homelessness due to common characteristics. This difference in how "homelessness" was defined may account for some of the differences in their findings, as may the fact that Rosenheck and Fontana's study included only men and was conducted nearly two decades before Washington and colleagues' study, which included only women. Both studies were observational, cross-sectional studies which could not examine causality, although Rosenheck and Fontana's structural equation model allowed for modeling of temporal relationships among some variables. A longitudinal study collecting baseline data prior to military service and tracking individuals through time to determine ever/never homeless outcomes would contribute greatly to the evidence base in this area.

No study identified in our review found a direct significant association between prolonged/intense combat exposure and homelessness. The definition of prolonged or intense combat exposure has varied, which increases the difficulty in evaluating existing evidence. The NVVRS examined both intensity and duration of combat.[44] It also found an association between PTSD and lower military pay-grade, which Seal[49] used as part of a proxy definition for combat exposure (along with branch of service and single vs. repeat deployment). Rosenheck and Fontana[15] found no direct association between homelessness and intense combat exposure, but they found direct effects of combat exposure on non-PTSD psychiatric illness (schizophrenia was not assessed), substance abuse, not being married, and low social support after discharge, all of which were associated with homelessness. They did find a weak association between homelessness and "participation in wartime atrocities,"[15] a uniquely regrettable military exposure; this measure has not been replicated by other studies. Research primarily comparing Vietnam-era and post-Vietnam era Veterans has found that Veterans most at risk for homelessness are in the age cohorts least likely to have served in combat.[58] Long-term, longitudinal research involving Veterans from OIF and OEF should be undertaken to reassess the role of combat and its associated risk for homelessness. The recent development of the Deployment Risk and Resilience Inventory (DRRI)[59] provides a multi-scale inventory capable of capturing data on more nuanced aspects of combat experience and associated stress, and which has been validated for use with OIF Veterans. Future research should consider the use of this inventory.

As previously mentioned, however, risk factors for homelessness rarely occur in isolation. For this reason, the conceptual attempt to understand Veteran homelessness requires acknowledgement of synergistic effects that may occur after exposure to multiple direct or indirect risk factors.

Combat's Impact on Mental Health

Clearly, not all mental health problems experienced by Veterans are related to their military service. Despite pre-service screening, some military service members will enter the military with mental health problems that may or may not be known at the time. As already discussed, childhood trauma, which frequently leads to mental health problems, has been shown to increase the risk of homelessness in both Veteran and general populations. Similarly, Rosenheck and Fontana's[15] finding that psychiatric treatment of any kind before the age of 18 increased the risk of homelessness among the 0.7 percent of Veterans in their sample receiving such treatment suggests that, for the small population affected, pre-existing mental health problems are likely to exert a significant and diverse influence on their well-being. Our focus here, however, is on mental illness that is more directly linked to military service, the best-studied example of which is combat-related PTSD. Estimates of lifetime PTSD expression within Veteran populations vary, but one recent national study of OEF/OIF Veterans entering VA care found a prevalence of 21.8 percent for PTSD, a notable portion of the 42.7 percent with any mental health diagnosis.[49]

PTSD, it should be noted, is more prevalent in the general population than is often assumed, and as one study[60] of incarcerated Veterans found, combat exposure may not be the type of trauma most strongly associated with developing PTSD, even among Veterans. As the literature on PTSD expands, there is an increasing acceptance that, at least in some cases, psychosocial context – the daily stresses individuals encounter – may be as important to the expression of PTSD symptoms as the severity of the original trauma.[61] Keeping these caveats in mind, several studies have consistently found an association between prolonged or intense combat exposure and an increased risk of a PTSD diagnosis, PTSD symptoms, and/or anxiety or depression, even when controlling for predisposing factors. The NVVRS report[44] as well as Rosenheck and Fontana's study based on the same data set[15] both found PTSD more prevalent among those who had served longer tours of duty and who reported higher "war zone stress" as measured by a variety of traumatic exposures. An association between combat exposure and PTSD has also been found by a longitudinal study that looked at twin pairs with discordant Vietnam theater/era service,[45,46] as well as cross-sectional studies of mixed Veteran cohorts receiving VA primary care[47], active duty and reserve Iraq Veterans[48,49] and combined Iraq/Afghanistan National Guard Veterans returning for a repeat deployment.[50]

However, the evidence linking PTSD to homelessness remains limited by the small number, small size and/or non-generalizable sampling methods of existing studies. Positive PTSD screening was found to be associated with homelessness by Washington, Yano and McGuire[36] but not by Rosenheck and Fontana,[15] where the authors concluded that PTSD's effect was likely to be accounted for by other psychiatric disorders with which it shared variance.[15] In general, analysis of the association between mental illness and Veteran homelessness is limited by the inconsistency of mental health conditions assessed across and within studies. For example, Washington, Yano and McGuire[36] found an association between positive PTSD/anxiety disorder screening and homelessness, but not positive depression screening or problem alcohol use, and schizophrenia was not assessed. The NVVRS did not assess participants for schizophrenia, a condition associated with homelessness in the general population.[15] Perhaps not surprisingly, given that the study's sample was of men seeking care for mental health issues, Tessler, Rosenhack and Gamache[55] did not find any significant difference between the Addiction Severity Index (ASI)-Psychiatric scores of Veteran and non-Veteran homeless men.

As several authors of the studies reviewed noted, the existential challenges of life as a homeless person are likely to negatively impact an individual's mental health, so cross-sectional studies of the prevalence of mental illnesses among the homeless are unlikely to provide definitive evidence on the extent to which mental illness affects one's risk for homelessness. There is consistent evidence from research on the general homeless population that indicates mental illness (schizophrenia, bipolar disorder, and depression) is associated with homelessness, including the duration of homelessness.[19, 62-64] There is some disagreement, however, as to whether mental illness itself increases the risk of homelessness.[65]

Combat's Impact on Income and Employment

While an association between unstable employment and/or low income and homelessness seems intuitive, few studies have examined the strength of these associations within Veteran homeless populations. Washington, Yano and McGuire[36] found that among female Veterans, homelessness was associated with being unemployed and being disabled. Rosenheck and Fontana[15] did not include NVVRS data on post-deployment employment, disability, or income in their analysis and so could draw no conclusions.

In a study analyzing data from multiple waves of the Panel Study of Income Dynamics between 1968 and 2003, MacLean[51] found that combat exposure (not further defined by intensity or duration) increased the rates of disability and unemployment among Veterans compared to non-combat Veterans, both in their early working years and throughout life. MacLean's analysis suggested a direct cumulative disadvantage effect that negatively affected combat Veterans regardless of pre-military service characteristics such as education. In contrast, Resnick and Rosenheck's[66] study of 5,862 male Veterans participating in a vocational rehabilitation program, the majority of whom reported being homeless, found that service in a theater of operations was associated with better chances of employment at program discharge. However, Veterans with PTSD or other severe mental illness were found to have less successful employment outcomes (fewer days worked), a finding consistent with other studies which have found negative correlations between severity of PTSD symptoms and wage levels/full-time employment[44, 47, 67, 68] and between PTSD diagnosis and stability of employment.[44]

Combat's Impact on Social Support

As among the general homeless population, low social support, though inconsistently defined, has been associated with Veteran homelessness. Rosenheck and Fontana[15] found that low social support in the year after discharge from the military had the strongest direct effect on homelessness risk. In bivariate analysis, the separate measure of not being married was also associated with an increased risk of homelessness, although the study design could not investigate whether homelessness preceded or followed not being (currently) married. Washington, Yano and McGuire[36] found that among female Veterans, marriage (a narrow but common measure of social support) was protective against homelessness.

Social support is a complex construct, and there is considerable academic discussion about the mechanisms through which social support actually makes a difference in people's lives, and what kinds of support matter most. Social support is by its nature located both within the individual's personal relationships (who may be married, have strong family ties, etc.) and the society around him or her (which may provide more institutional avenues for social support); when it is extended to consider one's relational position within society, and the opportunities for more institutional support, this is often conceptualized as social capital.[69, 70] All of the Veteran specific research studies identified defined social support predominantly in terms of individual relationships, with less attention paid to social capital/social support at the level of social institutions. None of the studies reviewed specifically investigated what type of social capital is most likely to provide support for homeless Veterans to move out of homelessness.

The only study identified which directly assessed associations between combat exposure and social support was the NVVRS,[44] which found an association between high war-zone stress (intense combat exposure) and poor family functioning, as well as more frequent divorce or marital problems. Several Department of Defense and other government agency reports have expressed concern at the impact that repeat or lengthy deployments may be having on the mental health of OEF/OIF troops,[71, 72] but this concern has been poorly translated into research on the psychosocial difficulties of post-deployment life. Some of the findings from the studies reviewed suggest that poor social support may also be associated with worse employment outcomes,[66] though the direction of the relationship is not clear. PTSD remains better researched than (re)adjustment disorders or employment difficulties, so the literature on PTSD provides the best source of data on combat's influence on social support.

Prolonged combat exposure increases the risk of developing PTSD, which the NVVRS found to be associated with extreme isolation and extreme unhappiness.[44] More recent studies have found an association between PTSD and poorer emotional well-being and poorer social functioning among Veterans.[73] A 2008 literature review[74] cited numerous studies finding PTSD negatively impacted family functioning, but its references to Veteran-specific literature were limited in both number and strength of findings. In contrast, Magruder and colleagues[47] did not find any association, in their random sample of male primary care patients at two VAMCs, between PTSD and social support (as measured by living alone or with someone). Rosenheck, Leda and Gallup,[75] in their analysis of 1988-1989 data from homeless male Veterans seeking residential treatment or intensive case management for mental illness, did not find any significant association between Veterans with "combat stress" (a measure defined using PTSD diagnostic criteria) and social adjustment as measured by marriage, employment or justice system history. However, the authors pointed out that this was likely to be a result of their sampling limitations, and that compared to the general population of Veterans at the time, the entire sample exhibited "severe social and vocational problems," suggesting the underlying impact of mental illness on multiple intermediate outcomes that might increase the risk of homelessness.

Some Exposures, Like Alcohol/Drug Abuse and Low Social Support, That May Increase Risk of Homelessness Frequently Emerge During Service or the Readjustment Period

Drug and/or alcohol abuse, though widely studied and popularly accepted as risk factors for homelessness, have not been consistently shown to increase the risk of homelessness among Veterans. There is limited evidence suggesting that alcohol and drug use increase the risk of homelessness, but there are many potential confounding factors. While exposure to these risk factors is not intrinsic to military service, evidence suggests that military culture and/or the inherently disruptive nature of military service tours increase the likelihood of negative outcomes for both alcohol/drug abuse and social support. These weak associations with the onset of alcohol/drug abuse and low social support post-service explain why "military service" in general is included in the conceptual model, even though in other ways (through employment and educational training, for example) military service may provide protection against homelessness.

A higher prevalence of problem alcohol use has been shown among Veterans compared to the general populations. Kulka et al. found that 40 percent of male Veterans had abused alcohol for some period in their lives, compared to 25 percent among male civilians.[44] While results varied by race and sex, the general finding of the NVVRS was that problem alcohol and substance use, though higher among both male and female Veterans than among the general population, was not higher among male Vietnam theater Veterans compared to male Vietnam era Veterans.[44] More recently, Erbes and colleagues, examining a small, self-selecting sample of OEF/OIF Veterans enrolling at a VAMC, found 27 percent reported current (as opposed to lifetime) hazardous drinking practices.[73]

Bray and Hourani[52] analyzed data from cross-sectional Department of Defense surveys of active duty service members conducted regularly between 1980 and 2005. Their analysis found that, despite earlier declines in heavy drinking in 2005, more than one in six active duty personnel were likely to be heavy drinkers.[52] These findings lend support to concerns cited by the authors that military culture, in contrast to its attitudes towards smoking and illicit drug use, remains permissive of problem alcohol use; the influence of this experience while in the military may shape post-service behavior. Arguably, rates of alcohol and drug use among active duty service members might reflect usage in the general population in their age cohort, especially for younger cohorts among whom substance use is generally believed to be highest. However, Bray and Hourani's analysis did control for socio-demographic trends on substance use and still found no decline.[52] More significantly, Jacobson and colleagues conducted a longitudinal study that collected baseline and post-deployment data on alcohol use, and found that the Reserve and National Guard personnel and younger service members who deployed with combat exposures were more likely to develop new problem alcohol use during the post-deployment period, and that this risk was greatest among those also diagnosed with PTSD or PTSD and depression.[53] This finding suggests an alternate concern: that problem alcohol use may be related not just to the immediate stresses or "culture" of military service but also to its after-effects. Rosenheck, Leda and Gallup[75] using data from homeless male Veterans seeking residential treatment in the late 1980s, had previously found an association (p<.02) between "combat stress" – defined by *Diagnostic and Statistical Manual of Mental Disorders, Fourth Edition* (DSM-IV) PTSD symptoms – and alcohol problems, along with a marginally significant association between combat stress and substance use. Similarly, Benda's (2006) study of Veterans seeking domiciliary care for substance abuse found a negative association between PTSD severity and the length of time before readmission. All of these findings highlight, again, the inter-connection of potential risk factors.

However, the evidence on the association between alcohol and/or drug use problems and homelessness is limited. Rosenheck and Fontana's analysis of NVVRS data[15] found that substance abuse, particularly alcohol abuse, had a direct effect on risk of homelessness. Tessler, Rosenheck and Gamache[55] found that homeless Veterans scored significantly higher on the ASI-Alcohol score than homeless non-Veterans, suggesting that alcohol problems may be more common to the experiences of homeless Veterans. The study found no significant difference in mean ASI-Drugs scores in the two populations, but did find younger Veteran cohorts (those born after 1953) scored significantly higher on the ASI-Drugs score than did older cohorts. Age is only one factor that may be of relevance in understanding differences in risk related to substance use within the homeless Veteran population. The NVVRS, for example, found that drug and alcohol abuse problems were most pronounced among Hispanic combat Veterans,[44] and another study that focused on homeless Native American Veterans[76] found they were more likely than other homeless Veterans to have an alcohol use problem, but less likely to have drug use problems (or a psychiatric diagnosis). Leda, Rosenheck and Gallup[77] found, among their sample of homeless mentally ill Veterans seeking treatment, that substance abuse diagnoses were less common among women than among men. Benda[78] found that, among a random sample of homeless male Veterans seeking domiciliary care, combat exposure was on a par with alcohol and drug abuse as a predictor for readmission for substance abuse treatment (HR 1.56-1.97 CI, p<.01); the female sample did not have sufficient combat exposure to test this association, but as Benda suggests, this is likely to have changed as more women are exposed to combat-like conditions.[78]

Military Sexual Trauma (MST) May Place Veterans at Increased Risk of Homelessness

Awareness of the problem of MST has increased dramatically in the past decade,[79] although evidence indicates that sexual harassment and assault, especially, but not only, directed against female service members occurred in earlier eras of service as well. A 1999 study of female VA outpatients found military sexual assault was reported by 23 percent of respondents;[80] another study from the 1990s of inpatient and randomly selected outpatient female Veterans at one VAMC similarly found that 14 percent of female Veterans under age 50 reported attempted rape during military service.[81] Kimerling's analysis of data from over 125,000 OEF/OIF Veterans, who are now routinely screened for MST, found a prevalence of 15.1 percent positive MST screening among women and 0.7 percent positive screening among men.[82]

The only study to date which has examined the association between MST and homelessness is Washington, Yano and McGuire's study of housed and non-housed female Veterans in the

Los Angeles area.[36] That study found that sexual assault during military service was associated with Veteran homelessness. Kimerling did not look at housing outcomes, but found significant associations between positive MST screening and PTSD diagnosis, other anxiety disorders, depression, adjustment disorder, substance disorder or alcohol disorder.[82] Benda's study constructed hazard models which indicated that sexual and physical abuse, regardless of when they occurred (in childhood or adulthood, during or after military service), were stronger predictors of readmission to substance abuse treatment for homeless female Veterans than for homeless male Veterans, who rarely reported military sexual or physical abuse.[78] Hankin and colleagues found that female Veterans who reported having ever experienced sexual assault were twice as likely to report current alcohol abuse and three times as likely to report symptoms of depression.[80] A 2003 literature review[83] studied mental service utilization among female Veterans and concluded that sexual trauma, whether service-related or not, was associated with PTSD. Murdoch and Nichol found that sexual harassment while in the military – which was experienced by 90 percent of female Veterans under age 50 in the sample – was significantly associated with an increased risk of anxiety, depression, and poorer general health on three different measures, all of which could contribute cumulatively to increased risk for homelessness.[81]

Sexual and physical abuse are probably under-reported both inside and outside of military settings, and given the fact that non-military related sexual abuse cannot be service-connected, there is an especial risk that it remains under-reported among Veterans.[83] It has been argued that female Veterans suffer from higher rates of PTSD than male soldiers and have experienced higher rates of sexual assault than the general population.[16] Experience with sexual assault has been linked to PTSD, depression, alcohol and drug abuse, disrupted social networks, and employment difficulties, all factors known to increase one's risk for homelessness.[16] The possibility that there is a cumulative effect of abuse on an individual's resiliency or well-being, coupled with poor confidence in rates of reporting, make it difficult to determine to what extent MST acts as an independent risk factor for homelessness. Given the range of associated outcomes, it may be that MST, like combat exposure, exerts greater influence on intermediate outcomes than on homelessness itself. Further research into the extent of MST's association with these outcomes is recommended.

KEY QUESTION #4. What is the relationship between incarceration and homelessness among Veterans?

After a steady rise in the number of Veterans in prison since 1985, the number, which peaked at about 153,100 in 2000, had declined by about nine percent to 140,000 by 2004.[84] The age adjusted incarceration rate for Veterans, which accounts for the older distribution of the Veteran population when compared to the general population, is about 1,253 per 100,000 or about 10 percent lower than the rate for non-Veterans. An older study of mentally ill Veterans found 15.7 percent had an incarceration history.[85] A more recent national study found three percent of Veterans were incarcerated.[86]

Incarcerated Veterans were more likely to have committed violent offenses than the incarcerated non-Veteran population.[84] Over half of Veterans serving in state prisons (57 percent), but fewer than half of non-Veterans (47 percent) were in prison for violent offenses. While about 20 percent of non-Veterans were incarcerated for homicide (12 percent) or rape/sexual assault (9 percent), over a third of Veterans were serving sentences for homicide (15 percent) and rape/sexual assault (23 percent). A similar pattern is found for active-duty personnel held in military prison. In 2004, 46 percent of all inmates in military custody were incarcerated for violent offenses, with rape or sexual assault being the most common reason for incarceration, accounting for 29 percent of inmates in military prisons.[84]

Incarcerated Veterans have also been found to have higher rates of drug abuse,[85, 87-89] treatment for mental health disorders,[85-87] and PTSD[87] than unincarcerated Veterans. On the other hand, incarcerated Veterans have comparable rates of alcohol abuse and mental health disorders, and lower rates of drug use than incarcerated non-Veterans.[84]

Finally, while Veterans in federal prison were twice as likely to be White, non-Hispanic (49 percent) as non-Veterans (24 percent), incarceration patterns for Veterans showed the same types of racial and ethnic disparities in imprisonment as in the general population. While the 2005-2007 American Community Survey estimated that 82 percent of Veterans were White, non-Hispanic, 10 percent Black, and 5 percent Hispanic in 2004; 49 percent of Veterans in federal prisons were White, non-Hispanic, 38 percent were Black, and 5 percent were Hispanic. In state prisons 54 percent of Veterans were White, 32 percent Black, and 6 percent Hispanic.[84]

Incarceration and Homelessness

In a review of the literature on incarceration and homelessness, Metraux and colleagues note the demographic similarities between homeless and incarcerated populations – both are typically poor, uneducated, and minority populations with few job skills – and suggest a bi-directional association between homelessness and incarceration.[90] They found that about 10 percent of those entering prison have a recent history of homelessness, and that at least 10 percent of those leaving prison experience some period of subsequent homelessness. In reviewing studies of the homeless, they found that as many as 20 percent of the adult homeless population is likely to have some lifetime experience of incarceration.

Metraux et al. found in their review of the literature that inmates of local jails, as opposed to state or federal prison inmates, had a cyclic pattern of homelessness and incarceration leading to prolonged residential instability. In contrast, because prisons are often located remotely from inmates' local communities, social ties that may be necessary to support successful integration upon release are often disrupted. Inmates of prison, therefore, are more likely to become homeless within 30 days of release.[90]

In exploring the factors associated with homelessness among the incarcerated, their review found shelter use prior to incarceration to be the strongest predictor of shelter use upon re-entry from prison. Other factors found to be associated with homelessness among the incarcerated include:

- **Ineffective discharge planning:** Prisons are generally remote from the communities to which prisoners will be returning, making access with local service agencies difficult;

- **Legal and regulatory restrictions**: Many laws limit access to public housing, drivers' licenses, and eligibility for government financial support programs;

- **Full sentencing laws:** Laws requiring sentence completion mean fewer prisoners are released on parole and probation, eliminating a source of support and supervision during the period of re-integration into the community; and

- **Financial instability:** Loss of job skills and reluctance of employers to hire former convicts can make it difficult to earn enough to make rent payments.[90]

In addition to factors that put prisoners at risk for subsequent homelessness, the review points to the "criminalization" of many of the activities of the homeless as factors increasing their risk for incarceration. This leads to what the review describes as an "'institutional circuit,' where a series of institutions provide sequential stints of housing in place of a stable, community-based living situation."[90]

Legal and Regulatory Barriers

A recently updated report by the Legal Action Center, *After Prison: Roadblocks to Reentry*,[91] describes the barriers faced by people with criminal records. Particularly for those with drug-related offenses, these barriers include restrictions on driving, limits on access to public assistance programs, and limits on access to public housing. Several studies have pointed to the impact of child support requirements on incarcerated parents, noting that incarcerated parents with child support obligations on average owe $10,000 upon entering prison, and owe on average $20,000 when released.[92,93] Minimum wage workers have little hope of making the typical monthly payment obligations of from $225 to $300 per month, often leading to further financial and legal difficulties. This problem is of particular relevance noting that in the most recent CHALENG report, legal assistance for child support was ranked as the second highest unmet need of responding homeless Veterans.[26]

Studies of Homelessness and Incarceration among Veterans

Very few studies have specifically investigated homelessness and incarceration in the Veteran population. The most salient feature of the literature is its sparseness. However, those few studies support the broader evidence that suggests that homelessness and incarceration have a bi-directional relationship.[90] Homelessness, through the criminalization of the activities of daily living while homeless, such as panhandling, vagrancy, trespassing, and public urination; and through criminal activities taken on either to cope with homelessness, such as alcohol and drug use, or to survive, such as stealing and prostitution, often leads to incarceration. Conversely, incarceration, by its separation from home communities and through legal restrictions on re-integration with those communities, often puts individuals at risk for homelessness upon release.

A 2003 study assessed whether substance abuse and psychiatric illness are related to offenses, and attempted to identify the strongest predictors of and protective factors against criminal offenses among homeless Veterans with substance abuse problems (n = 188).[94] Measures included the Addiction Severity Index (ASI); the Multi-Problem Screening Inventory (MPSI); the Multidimensional Scale of Perceived Social Support; the Self-Efficacy Scale; and the Ego Identity Scale. Respondents were found to be representative of the population from which they were drawn. Half were White, about 40 percent were Black, and most had lived in a rural area during adolescence; and there were high levels of depression and suicidality. One-third (33 percent) reported no offenses in the past year and 41 percent reported committing multiple offenses. Alcohol abuse (OR = 2.04, 95% CI = 1.80, 2.30), drug abuse (OR = 3.57, 95% CI = 3.01, 4.05), and number of prior psychiatric hospitalizations (OR = 1.27, 95% CI = 1.15, 1.39) were significantly associated with committing a crime in the past year, while depression and suicidal thoughts were not. In a separate analysis, those sexually abused before age 18 were two and a half times more likely to have committed a crime in the past year (OR = 2.50, 95% CI = 2.33, 2.70). On the other hand, those with a strong sense of self-efficacy, resilience, or ego-integrity were significantly less likely to have committed a crime in the past year (OR = 0.28, 95% CI = 0.17, 0.41; OR = 0.32, 95% CI = 0.20, 0.47; OR = 0.48, 95% CI = 0.40, 0.58, respectively). Those who reported usual, full-time employment in the previous three years were about half as likely to have committed a crime in the previous year (OR = 0.46, 95% CI = 0.30, 0.61) and higher levels of education were associated with lower likelihood of committing a crime (OR = 0.57, 95% CI = 0.43, 0.71). The authors suggest that in homeless Veterans who abuse substances, co-morbid mental health problems may increase the likelihood of incarceration; but that even among this population, a strong sense of self-efficacy, resilience, and ego-integrity can reduce the likelihood of incarceration.[94]

A study of patients with serious mental health disorders recruited from a VA mental institution found that lifetime homelessness was most strongly associated with lifetime history of incarceration (OR = 4.36, 95% CI = 2.73, 6.94) but was also associated with lower levels of treatment adherence (OR = 0.80, 95% CI = 0.66, 0.96); that recent homelessness (in the previous four weeks) was strongly associated with recent incarceration (OR = 26.41, 95% CI = 5.23, 133.4); and those who had any lifetime experience of homelessness were four times more likely to have a lifetime history of incarceration (OR = 4.24, 95% CI = 2.67, 6.71). While the authors note that these findings suggest a strong bi-directional association of homelessness and incarceration, the findings may not be generalizable beyond VA patients with bipolar disorders.[95]

A small study (n= 62) evaluated self-selected, mentally ill Veteran inmates who were either homeless at the time of arrest or anticipated being homeless after release.[96] Most were Black (74 percent) and unmarried (89 percent). Over a quarter (26 percent) were homeless at the time of arrest, and three-quarters (75 percent) had had a prior episode of homelessness. Nearly all subjects (94 percent) reported a prior arrest and 73 percent were being detained on felony charges. The primary psychiatric diagnoses were schizophrenia (37 percent), mood disorders (35 percent), PTSD (5 percent), adjustment disorders (5 percent), and pedophilia (3 percent). Eighty-three percent reported either a diagnosis of substance abuse disorder or significant problems with alcohol and drugs, and 76 percent reported a history of prior psychiatric hospitalization. The authors suggest the study shows that large urban jails may be useful locations for outreach to mentally ill, homeless Veterans.[96]

Jail Diversion Programs for Veterans

Because of the strong association between homelessness and incarceration, interventions that divert offenders from prison have been seen by some as promising approaches both to limit the direct negative effects of incarceration and to mitigate the association of incarceration with subsequent homelessness. The literature on diversion programs specifically targeting Veterans is very sparse, as such programs are relatively new. However, more general diversion programs have a long history dating back to the 1970s, and there is a large body of literature both describing and evaluating the effectiveness of these programs. A comprehensive and systematic review of that literature is beyond the scope of this review. However, because of the potential importance of these programs in addressing issues of homelessness, we provide a brief overview of the various types of diversion programs that have been developed.

Broadly, diversion programs fall into two categories, pre-booking vs. post-booking diversion. In pre-booking programs, individuals are diverted prior to arrest, often through the discretion and decision of specially trained police. In post-booking programs, individuals are diverted after arrest but before prosecution and incarceration, and the program is generally overseen by the court. This review will focus on post-booking programs, as they are generally the more formal programs and the better-studied.

Post-booking programs operate either out of standard criminal courts or out of specialty courts that target specific types of offenders such as the mentally ill, drug users and, more recently, Veterans. Early diversion programs focused on diverting mentally ill offenders from jail and towards treatment options with a goal to reducing jail time and recidivism, and providing effective mental health treatment. In an early survey of jail diversion programs for the mentally ill, Steadman and colleagues provided a definition of jail diversion programs as "specific (formal or informal) programs that *screen* defined groups of detainees for the presence of mental disorder; use mental health professionals to *evaluate* all those detainees identified in the screening; and *negotiate* with prosecutors, defense attorneys, community-based mental health providers, and the courts to produce a mental health disposition outside the jail in lieu of prosecution or as a condition of a reduction in charges (whether or not a formal conviction occurs)" (italics in the original).[97]

In 1995, the SAMHSA established the National GAINS Center as a locus for the collection and dissemination of information on effective mental health and substance abuse programs for individuals with co-occurring disorders who come into contact with the justice system (web site at: http://gainscenter.samhsa.gov/html). Between 2002 and 2007, through its Center for Mental Health Services (CMHS), SAMHSA provided Targeted Capacity Expansion (TCE) grants to support the development of evidence-based jail diversion programs. This funding only supported programs that operated out of traditional court programs; funding could not support programs operating out of specialty courts. With recognition of the increasing number of combat Veterans returning from overseas with PTSD and of the associated risk for involvement with the criminal justice system, in 2008, CMHS began funding a Jail Diversion and Trauma Recovery Program to support implementation and expansion of jail diversion programs specifically for individuals with PTSD and other trauma-related disorders, providing prioritized eligibility for Veterans. Since 2008, CMHS has awarded 13 grants through this program. All programs have specific and similar requirements for program evaluation and standard data elements for collection.

A national multi-site evaluation of the programs funded through the TCE grants found mixed results among the programs and overall. The most consistent effect was an increase in service utilization, with diversion being associated with increases in counseling, mental health hospitalizations, emergency room use, and use of mental health medications. However, this effect was found, in general, to decrease in time with service utilization, being lower at the 12-month follow-up period than at three months. In addition, while differences in access to and quantity of treatment were significant, treatment intensity in both groups, diverted and non-diverted, were low.[98] Findings were mixed for changes in drug and alcohol use, with some sites showing decreased use while others showed increased use for both drug and alcohol use, and there was little evidence of effectiveness on mental health outcomes or quality of life. Across all sites, diversion programs resulted in significant increases in days at risk (not institutionalized) and days in the community, and fewer days in jail. However, there was no change in recidivism.

The findings from this study are consistent with the findings of other studies and reviews.[99-103] Some care should be taken in interpreting these findings as studies varied in quality and there was substantial variation in the characteristics of the programs evaluated. Nevertheless, the lack of significant findings on a number of outcomes and the consistency of findings related to criminal justice outcomes suggests that what biases there were likely did not act to overestimate the effectiveness of these programs. If true, these findings suggest that while diversion programs may not be effective in treating the mental health needs of the participants, that from a public policy and safety perspective, diversion programs can lead to reduced days in jail and increased days in the community without increasing risks for public safety.

Finally, with regard to issues related to homelessness, one evaluation of these same programs found that consistent housing throughout the 12-month study period was the factor most strongly associated with post-enrollment arrests. The only other factors significantly associated with no vs. any post-enrollment arrest was prior arrests and number of prior jail days.[99] These findings underscore the importance of stable housing for successful diversion programs.

Mental Health and Drug Courts

While many of the earlier programs and their evaluations were limited to diversion programs overseen by the traditional court system, later programs, in an attempt to enhance program effectiveness, developed a model of specialty mental health and drug courts which sought to bring together the experts and resources needed for effective oversight and treatment of these detainees. In his review of studies of diversion programs for persons with mental illness, Sirotich[101] looked at six studies in which diversion programs were overseen by mental health courts. Similar to the findings for non-specialty courts, Sirotich found inconsistent results among the programs supervised by mental health courts, with the most consistent finding being that divertees showed no increase in the number of jail days relative to those not diverted; two studies reported a decrease in jail time for mental health court participants but not for those receiving treatment as usual; and two studies reported no change in jail time for either group.[101] Finally, in a review of drug court effects on recidivism, Wilson and colleagues found offenders participating in drug courts less likely to re-offend than those treated with traditional justice programs.[104] That review found weak evidence that effectiveness varied by the specific drug court model employed. Programs that dismissed charges or expunged records appeared to be more successful than those in which the incentives for successful completion were more ambiguous. Programs that used a single treatment provider appeared slightly more successful than those providing treatment by multiple providers. Regardless of model, studies were inconclusive as to whether effectiveness would persist after the individual left the program.

Veterans Courts

Noting an increase in the number of Veterans appearing in court for criminal offenses often related to substance abuse and mental health disorders, and building on the models of mental health and drug courts, a number of jurisdictions have begun to develop Veterans Courts. The first such court was established in Anchorage, Alaska in 2004[105] to provide an alternative to jail time for Veterans charged with misdemeanors. In 2009, Judge Robert T. Russell described the 10 Key Components of the Veterans Treatment Court of Buffalo, New York, which was established in January 2008. These components were modeled on the key components of drug courts as described by the U.S. Department of Justice.[106] As noted above, it was about that time that SAMHSA began funding to support Jail Diversion and Trauma Recovery Programs with priority for program eligibility given to Veterans. That program now provides support and technical assistance to programs in 13 states, including Colorado, Connecticut, Georgia, Illinois, Massachusetts, and Vermont (funded in 2008); Florida, North Carolina, New Mexico, Ohio, Rhode Island and Texas (funded in 2009); and Pennsylvania (funded in 2010). Veterans Courts have also been established in Tulsa, Oklahoma and Nevada; and California law allows the court to grant special consideration to anyone who alleges that he or she has committed an offense as a result of sexual trauma, traumatic brain injury, PTSD, substance abuse, or a mental health problem as a result of military service.[107] In addition, a Department of Veterans Affairs Information Letter reported that as of April 2009 more than one third of VAMCs indicated that they currently engaged or intended to engage with local justice system partners to coordinate services for justice-involved Veterans.[108] Likely because these programs are new, we have found no studies evaluating their effectiveness.

Veterans leaving prison are at high risk for homelessness because of the many social and legal barriers to re-integration. That makes prisons a good place to do outreach to Veterans at risk for homelessness. However, to address the problem will require a multi-modal approach that brings together the corrections agencies responsible for releasing the Veteran, the justice system responsible for parole or probationary oversight, the mental health system in the community where the Veteran will be released to help address any psychiatric and substance use problems, the local VA and Veterans Health Administration (VHA) agencies, and the local housing agencies to help link the Veteran to housing or supportive housing as needed. This will require not only developing new collaborative approaches, but also sponsoring research on ways in which these collaborations (and which types of collaborations) can most effectively reduce the likelihood of homelessness upon re-entry, including developing a better understanding of how to identify those most at risk for homelessness post-release.

Conversely, homeless Veterans are at risk for imprisonment because of the criminalization of the activities of daily living while homeless, and as a result of activities to help cope and survive while homeless. To break the cycle of homelessness⇒incarceration⇒homelessness, the VA should encourage research on Veterans Courts to determine how to implement them so as to effectively divert already homeless Veterans (or Veterans at risk for homelessness because of criminal activities) from increasing their risk for continued (or new) homelessness by creating opportunities to avoid prison and the negative consequences deriving from both a criminal record and incarceration.

SUMMARY AND DISCUSSION

Our review of the evidence suggests that there is no easily generalizable path into homelessness. Both Veteran and non-Veteran homeless individuals are more likely than those in the general population to have been exposed to one or more risk factors such as childhood instability or trauma, mental illness, alcohol or substance abuse, chronic illness, low social support in adulthood, and low or unstable income. However, the precise strength of the association of each of these factors with the outcome of homelessness remains poorly measured, both for the Veteran homeless population as a whole and for sub-populations of interest such as women Veterans. This is due in part to the lack of studies designed to examine the directionality of relationships of these variables to the outcome of homelessness, but also in part to the inherently complex process of becoming homeless, which occurs as the result of multiple influences (both structural and individual), each with various potential moments of intervention.

While homeless Veterans are exposed to much the same broadly defined risk factors as other homeless individuals, the qualitative nature of those exposures will in some cases be different because of Veterans' experiences during military service or during the post-deployment period. The conceptual model developed for this report is a first step in identifying areas where we need to gather stronger evidence in order to understand how the unique experiences of Veterans, such as combat exposure or readjustment difficulty, might be contributing to their risk of experiencing other more generally shared risk factors for homelessness such as low or unstable income.

Veteran homelessness is unique in that some factors generally believed to be protective, such as being better educated or having better social support, do not appear to have quite the same protective efficacy in the Veteran population. While we have speculated in this report that their experiences as Veterans might somehow actively work against the protective value associated with these factors in other populations, this is an area which has not been adequately researched and where longitudinal research employing mixed methods would be of great value in substantiating or refuting such a hypothesis.

Veterans become separated from their normative communities in different ways: physically, through enlistment in the military or incarceration in jail or prison, and socially and culturally through mental illness, substance abuse, and disability. Each presents its own challenges for re-entry into and re-integration with support networks in former communities. The Veteran "advantage" in better social support is hypothesized on the basis of repeated measures of higher rates of ever-marriage, but as other authors have pointed out, this may not be the most meaningful measure of social support in this context. It is possible that the additional financial and emotional responsibilities of supporting a spouse and dependents may, under certain circumstances, actually enhance the risk of homelessness. As with education, however, higher levels of social support among homeless Veterans as compared to homeless non-Veterans does not appear to offer protection against homelessness.

While recent trends in the number of Veteran homeless are encouraging, studies suggesting that lowered recruitment standards may be related to the increase in homelessness among Veterans of the early all volunteer force should, if true, make us alert to a potential increase in homelessness among Operation Iraqi Freedom (OIF)/Operation Enduring Freedom (OEF) Veterans who were similarly recruited with lowered standards.[109, 110]

As mentioned in the introduction, ending homelessness entails the two distinct tasks of relieving homelessness among those who currently lack housing, and preventing the occurrence of homelessness among those at risk. The existing evidence illustrates in many ways the methodological difficulties inherent in identifying risk factors, such as mental illness, in a population where the condition of interest (homelessness) is likely to produce the risk factor. Causal links between many individual level factors and homelessness have not been well-established in the literature, and there may be a bi-directional relationship between homelessness and risk factors such as mental illness, substance abuse and incarceration. Moreover, given that homelessness may not occur for many years after deployment, targeting military level risk factors may be difficult, especially during the post-deployment period. It may be important to repeatedly engage and evaluate Veterans both qualitatively and quantitatively for years after service. Large-scale, long-term longitudinal studies, such as the Department of Defense Millenium Cohort Study, provide important opportunities for this type of research.[31] Furthermore, an assessment of a given Veteran's risk for homelessness will be incomplete if only individual level risk factors are evaluated. The structural level risk factors of the environment (affordable housing, employment opportunities) into which a Veteran has re-integrated need to be assessed as these are likely to contribute to the homelessness risk milieu.

RECOMMENDATIONS FOR FUTURE RESEARCH

This report identifies a number of gaps in the literature and makes key suggestions to define the agenda for future research on Veteran homelessness:

- Longitudinal studies with Operation Enduring Freedom (OEF)/Operation Iraqi Freedom (OIF) Veterans are needed to capture data on exposures occurring before homelessness occurs. Given the VA's current policy of pro-active enrollment and engagement of this cohort, opportunities exist to conduct longitudinal studies that collect information on all of the risk factors identified in this report. This research should control for structural risk factors such as housing market costs and available assistance programs.

- Longitudinal studies with all new cohorts of enlisting military service members could better determine the pre-existing presence of risk factors, such as low social support, alcohol or substance abuse problems, before military service. Policies should be developed to facilitate the use of data from enlistment screenings in research.

- Qualitative studies employing longitudinal, ethnographic methods to investigate the distinct experiences of homeless Veterans will help researchers to understand what is unique about Veteran exposure to risk factors common to the general homeless population. This remains poorly understood at present but may have important implications for designing homelessness prevention programs that will be effective for Veterans.

- Current research suggests that risk for violent criminal behavior varies by service branch. Research to confirm these differences and how to identify individuals at risk for continued post-military violent criminal behavior may help target interventions to those most at risk for post-military incarceration.

- Research on the post-deployment period is needed, with a particular focus on risk factors for loss of income and social support during this transition period, as well as rates of short-term homelessness experienced during this period. These data could be collected as part of longitudinal studies looking for relationships between short-term and more chronic homelessness in the longer term, which has been the focus of past research.

- Further research on military sexual trauma (MST), its relationship to homelessness, and appropriate MST prevention and treatment programs, is recommended.

- Research on Veterans Courts and other specialty courts should be continued in order to improve their performance and find effective alternatives to incarceration for Veterans.

- Systems perspective research on collaborations among Departments of Corrections, the VA, the Department of Housing and Urban Development (HUD), and local community health agencies could inform efforts to reduce the likelihood of homelessness upon re-entry from incarceration, including developing a better understanding of how to identify those most at risk for homelessness post-release.

- Most of the measures used to assess risk factors and personal characteristics of the homeless, including measures of substance abuse, mental health, and measures of social support, have been developed and normed on populations very different from the homeless. The applicability of these measures to homeless populations is unknown. Research should be undertaken to assess the applicability of these measures and to modify or develop new measures where warranted. Similarly, better defined research on the aspects of social support most relevant to improving Veterans' post-deployment adjustment would contribute both to addressing Veteran homelessness and the literature's broader understanding of the function of social support.

- Long-term studies repeatedly collecting both quantitative and qualitative data, though always relatively difficult and costly to conduct, would greatly improve our understanding of Veterans' difficulties in re-engagement and re-integration over long periods of time after deployment, not just in the initial post-deployment year which is more frequently studied.

- Studies that include both individual and structural risk factors should be conducted to assess both their independent and contingent effects.

- Research is needed to investigate the relationship between the unique Veteran experience of "family readjustment difficulties" in the post-deployment period and other, more generalized concepts such as social support, as well as the relationship between family readjustment difficulties and clinical diagnoses of mental illness.

- To our knowledge, the direct relationship between injury/disability and increased risk of homelessness has not been well studied in the Veteran population. There is a need for research designed to examine injury as a risk factor for homelessness, both directly and indirectly, and taking into account the complex effects of serious injury on both income and quality of life/well-being.

REFERENCES

1. Homeless on Veterans Day. The New York Times. November 11, 2009.

2. US Interagency Council on Homelessness. Opening Doors, Federal Strategic Plan to Prevent and End Homelessness 2010.

3. Elliott M, Krivo LJ. Structural Determinants of Homelessness in the United States. Social Problems. 1991;38(1):113-31.

4. Ji E-G. A study of the structural risk factors of homelessness in 52 metropolitan areas in the United States. Int Socl Work. 2006;49(1):107-17.

5. Lee BA, PriceSpratlen T, Kanan JW. Determinants of Homelessness in Metropolitan Areas. Journal of Urban Affairs. [10.1111/1467-9906.00168]. 2003;25(3):335-56.

6. O'Connell MJ, Kasprow W, Rosenheck RA. Rates and risk factors for homelessness after successful housing in a sample of formerly homeless veterans. Psychiatr Serv. 2008 Mar;59(3):268-75.

7. Shinn M, Weitzman BC, Stojanovic D, Knickman JR, Jimenez L, Duchon L, et al. Predictors of homelessness among families in New York City: from shelter request to housing stability. American Journal of Public Health. [Research Support, Non-U.S. Gov't Research Support, U.S. Gov't, P.H.S.]. 1998 Nov;88(11):1651-7.

8. Koegel P, Burnam MA, Baumohl J. The causes of homelessness. In: Baumohl J, editor. Homelessness in America. Phoenix: The Oryx Press; 1996. p. 24-33.

9. DeCrappeo M, Pelletiere D, Crowley S, Teater E. Renters in the great recession, the crisis continues: National Low Income Housing Coalition. 2010 June.

10. Daskal J. In search of shelter: The growing shortage of affordable rental housing. Washington, DC: Center on Budget and Policy Priorities. 1998.

11. National Coalition for the Homeless. Why Are People Homeless? July 2009.

12. Pelletierre D. The rental housing affordability gap: Comparison of 2001 and 2003 American Housing Surveys: National Low Income Housing Coalition. 2006 March.

13. Dolbeare C. Housing policy: A general consideration. In: Baumohl J, editor. Homelessnes in America. Phoenix: The Oryx Press; 1996. p. 34-45.

14. The 2009 Annual Homeless Assessment Report to Congress: Office of Community Planning and Development, U.S. Department of Housing and Urban Development. June 2010.

15. Rosenheck R, Fontana A. A model of homelessness among male veterans of the Vietnam War generation. Am J Psychiatry. 1994 Mar;151(3):421-7.

16. Perl L. Veterans and Homelessness: Congressional Research Service. 2009 June 26, 2009.

17. Dietz TL. Predictors of reported current and lifetime substance abuse problems among a national sample of U.S. homeless. Subst Use Misuse. 2007;42(11):1745-66.

18. Johnson TP, Fendrich M, Johnson TP, Fendrich M. Homelessness and drug use: evidence from a community sample. Am J Prev Med. [Research Support, N.I.H., Extramural]. 2007 Jun;32(6 Suppl):S211-8.

19. Susser E, Moore R, Link B. Risk factors for homelessness. Epidemiol Rev. [Review]. 1993;15(2):546-56.

20. Fischer P, Breakey W. The epidemiology of alcohol, drug, and mental disorders among homeless persons. Am Psychol. 1991;46(11):1115-28.

21. Shelton KH, Taylor PJ, Bonner A, van den Bree M, Shelton KH, Taylor PJ, et al. Risk factors for homelessness: evidence from a population-based study. Psychiatric Services. [Research Support, N.I.H., Extramural]. 2009 Apr;60(4):465-72.

22. Johnson TP, Freels SA, Parsons JA, Vangeest JB. Substance abuse and homelessness: social selection or social adaptation? Addiction. [Research Support, Non-U.S. Gov't]. 1997 Apr;92(4):437-45.

23. Phelan JC, Link BG. Who are "the homeless"? Reconsidering the stability and composition of the homeless population. American Journal of Public Health. [Research Support, U.S. Gov't, P.H.S. Review]. 1999 Sep;89(9):1334-8.

24. Snow DA, Anderson L, Koegel P. Distorting Tendencies in Research on the Homeless. American Behavioral Scientist. 1994;37(4):15-.

25. Cackley AP, Schmidt P, Barry NS, Boggs K, Burnett R, Chatlos W, et al. Homelessness: A common vocabulary could help agencies collaborate and collect more consistent data: United States Government Accountability Office. 2010.

26. Kuhn JH, Nakashima J. The Sixteenth Annual Progress Report: Community Homelessness Assessment, Local Education and Networking Group for Veterans - Services for homeless veterans assessment and coordination: Community Homelessness Assessment, Local Education and Networking Group for Veterans. 2010 March 17.

27. Veteran Homelessness: A Supplemental Report to the 2009 Annual Homeless Assessment Report to Congress: Office of Community Planning and Development, U.S. Department of Housing and Urban Development and the U.S. Department of Veteran Affairs. January 2011.

28. Farrell BS, Gosling TW, Keisling SE, Nalwalk KM, Petrucci S, Shoemaker LL. Military personnel: Active duty benefits reflect changing demographics, but opportunities exist to improve United States Government Accountability Office. 2002.

29. Stewart DB. Military personnel: Active duty benefits reflect changing demographics, but continued focus is needed United States Government Accountability Office. 2002.

30. Health ViEWS: Health of Vietnam Era Women's Study. 2011 [cited 2011 March 9, 2011]; Available from: http://www.research.va.gov/programs/csp/csp579.cfm.

31. The Millenium Cohort Study. 2011 [cited 2011 March 9, 2011]; Available from: http://www.millenniumcohort.org/index.php.

32. Link B, Phelan J, Bresnahan M, Stueve A, Moore R, Susser E. Lifetime and five-year prevalence of homelessness in the United States: new evidence on an old debate. American Journal of Orthopsychiatry. [Research Support, U.S. Gov't, P.H.S.]. 1995 Jul;65(3):347-54.

33. Cunningham M, Henry M, Lyons W. Vital mission - Ending homelessness among veterans: National Alliance to End Homelessness. 2007 November.

34. Institute of Medicine Committee on the Initial Assessment of Readjustment Needs of Military Personnel V, Their F. Returning home from Iraq and Afghanistan: Preliminary assessment of readjustment needs of veterans, service members and their families. 2010.

35. Winkleby MA, Fleshin D. Physical, addictive, and psychiatric disorders among homeless veterans and nonveterans. Public Health Rep. 1993 Jan-Feb;108(1):30-6.

36. Washington D, Yano EM, McGuire J. Risk factors for homelessness among women veterans. Journal of Health Care for the Poor and Underserved. 2010 February 2010;21:82-91.

37. O'Toole TP, Conde-Martel A, Gibbon JL, Hanusa BH, Fine MJ. Health care of homeless veterans. J Gen Intern Med. 2003 Nov;18(11):929-33.

38. Wenzel SL, Gelberg L, Bakhtiar L, Caskey N, Hardie E, Redford C, et al. Indicators of chronic homelessness among veterans. Hosp Community Psychiatry. 1993 Dec;44(12):1172-6.

39. Adams J, Rosenheck R, Gee L, Seibyl CL, Kushel M. Hospitalized younger: a comparison of a national sample of homeless and housed inpatient veterans. J Health Care Poor Underserved. 2007 Feb;18(1):173-84.

40. Koegel P, Melamid E, Burnam MA. Childhood risk factors for homelessness among homeless adults. Am J Public Health. [Research Support, U.S. Gov't, P.H.S.]. 1995 Dec;85(12):1642-9.

41. Susser ES, Lin SP, Conover SA, Struening EL. Childhood antecedents of homelessness in psychiatric patients. American Journal of Psychiatry. [Research Support, Non-U.S. Gov't]. 1991 Aug;148(8):1026-30.

42. Rosenheck R, Koegel P. Characteristics of veterans and nonveterans in three samples of homeless men. Hosp Community Psychiatry. 1993 Sep;44(9):858-63.

43. Department of Defense Task Force on Mental Health. An achievable vision: Report of the Department of Defense Task Force on Mental Health. Falls Church, VA: Defense Health Board. 2007.

44. Kulka R, Schlenger W, Fairbank J, Hough R, Jordan B. Trauma and the Vietnam War generation: report of the findings from the National Vietnam Veterans Readjustment Study. New York: Brunner/Mazel; 1990.

45. Goldberg J, True W, Eisen S, Henderson W. A twin study of the effects of the Vietnam War on Posttraumatic Stress Disorder. Journal of the American Medical Association. 1990;263(9):1227-32.

46. Roy-Byrne P, Arguelles L, Vitek ME, Goldberg J, Keane TM, True WR, et al. Persistence and change of PTSD symptomatology--a longitudinal co-twin control analysis of the Vietnam Era Twin Registry. Social Psychiatry & Psychiatric Epidemiology. [Research Support, U.S. Gov't, Non-P.H.S. Research Support, U.S. Gov't, P.H.S. Twin Study]. 2004 Sep;39(9):681-5.

47. Magruder KM, Frueh BC, Knapp RG, Johnson MR, Vaughan JA, 3rd, Carson TC, et al. PTSD symptoms, demographic characteristics, and functional status among veterans treated in VA primary care clinics. Journal of Traumatic Stress. [Research Support, U.S. Gov't, Non-P.H.S.]. 2004 Aug;17(4):293-301.

48. Hoge CW, Auchterlonie JL, Milliken CS, Hoge CW, Auchterlonie JL, Milliken CS. Mental health problems, use of mental health services, and attrition from military service after returning from deployment to Iraq or Afghanistan. Jama. [Research Support, U.S. Gov't, Non-P.H.S.]. 2006 Mar 1;295(9):1023-32.

49. Seal KH, Metzler TJ, Gima KS, Bertenthal D, Maguen S, Marmar CR, et al. Trends and risk factors for mental health diagnoses among Iraq and Afghanistan veterans using Department of Veterans Affairs health care, 2002-2008. American Journal of Public Health. [Research Support, Non-U.S. Gov't Research Support, U.S. Gov't, Non-P.H.S.]. 2009 Sep;99(9):1651-8.

50. Polusny MA, Erbes CR, Arbisi PA, Thuras P, Kehle SM, Rath M, et al. Impact of prior Operation Enduring Freedom/Operation Iraqi Freedom combat duty on mental health in a predeployment cohort of National Guard soldiers. Military Medicine. [Research Support, Non-U.S. Gov't Research Support, U.S. Gov't, Non-P.H.S.]. 2009 Apr;174(4):353-7.

51. Maclean A. The things they carry: combat, disability and employment among U.S. men. Am Sociol Rev. 2010;75(4):563-85.

52. Bray R, Hourani L. Substance use trends among active duty military personnel: findings from the United States Department of Defense Health Related Behavior Surveys, 1980-2005: US Department of Defense. 2007. Report No.: Addiction 102.

53. Jacobson IG, Ryan MA, Hooper TI, Smith TC, Amoroso PJ, Boyko EJ, et al. Alcohol use and alcohol-related problems before and after military combat deployment. Jama. [Research Support, N.I.H., Extramural Research Support, U.S. Gov't, Non-P.H.S.]. 2008 Aug 13;300(6):663-75.

54. Rosenheck R, Kasprow W, Frisman L, Liu-Mares W. Cost-effectiveness of supported housing for homeless persons with mental illness. Arch Gen Psychiatry. 2003 Sep;60(9):940-51.

55. Tessler R, Rosenheck R, Gamache G. Comparison of homeless veterans with other homeless men in a large clinical outreach program. Psychiatr Q. 2002 Summer;73(2):109-19.

56. Sherbourne CD, Stewart AL. The MOS social support survey. Soc Sci Med. 1991;32(6):705-14.

57. Lin N, Dean A, Ensel WM. Social support, life events, and depression: Academic Pr; 1986.

58. Rosenheck R, Frisman L, Chung AM. The proportion of veterans among homeless men. Am J Public Health. 1994 Mar;84(3):466-9.

59. Vogt DS, Proctor SP, King DW, King LA, Vasterling JJ. Validation of scales from the Deployment Risk and Resilience Inventory in a sample of Operation Iraqi Freedom veterans. Assessment. 2008 Dec;15(4):391-403.

60. Saxon AJ, Davis TM, Sloan KL, McKnight KM, McFall ME, Kivlahan DR. Trauma, Symptoms of Posttraumatic Stress Disorder, and Associated Problems Among Incarcerated Veterans. Psychiatr Serv. [10.1176/appi.ps.52.7.959]. 2001;52(7):959-64.

61. Miller KE, Rasmussen A. War exposure, daily stressors, and mental health in conflict and post-conflict settings: Bridging the divide between trauma-focused and psychosocial frameworks. Social Science & Medicine. [10.1016/j.socscimed.2009.09.029]. 2010;70(1):7-16.

62. Koegel P, Burnam MA. Alcoholism among homeless adults in the inner city of Los Angeles. Archives of General Psychiatry. [Comparative Study Research Support, Non-U.S. Gov't Research Support, U.S. Gov't, P.H.S.]. 1988 Nov;45(11):1011-8.

63. Folsom D, Jeste DV. Schizophrenia in homeless persons: a systematic review of the literature. Acta Psychiatr Scand. 2002 Jun;105(6):404-13.

64. Reardon ML, Burns AB, Preist R, Sachs-Ericsson N, Lang AR. Alcohol use and other psychiatric disorders in the formerly homeless and never homeless: Prevalence, age of onset, comorbidity, temporal sequencing, and service utilization. Substance Use & Misuse. 2003;38(3-6):601-44.

65. Sullivan G, burnam A, Koegel P. Pathways to homelessness among the mentally ill. Soc Psychiatry Psychiatr Epidemiol. 2000;35:444-50.

66. Resnick SG, Rosenheck RA. Posttraumatic stress disorder and employment in veterans participating in Veterans Health Administration Compensated Work Therapy. J Rehabil Res Dev. 2008;45(3):427-35.

67. Smith MW, Schnurr PP, Rosenheck RA, Smith MW, Schnurr PP, Rosenheck RA. Employment outcomes and PTSD symptom severity. Mental Health Services Research. [Comparative Study Research Support, U.S. Gov't, Non-P.H.S.]. 2005 Jun;7(2):89-101.

68. Savoca E, Rosenheck R. The civilian labor market experiences of Vietnam-era veterans: The influence of psychiatric disorders. J Men Health Policy Econ. 2000;3(4):199-207.

69. Harpham T, Grant E, Thomas E. Measuring social capital within health surveys: key issues. Health Policy Plan. 2002 Mar;17(1):106-11.

70. Irwin J, LaGory M, Ritchey F, Fitzpatrick K. Social assets and mental distress among the homeless: Exploring the roles of social support and other forms of social capital on depression. Social Science & Medicine. [10.1016/j.socscimed.2008.09.008]. 2008;67(12):1935-43.

71. An Achievable Vision: Report of the Department of Defense Task Force on Mental Health: U.S. Department of Defense. 2007.

72. Committee on the Initial Assessment of Readjustment Needs of Military Personnel V, Their F, Board on the Health of Selected P, Institute of M. Returning Home from Iraq and Afghanistan: Preliminary Assessment of Readjustment Needs of Veterans, Service Members, and Their Families. Washington, D.C.: The National Academies Press; 2010.

73. Erbes C, Westermeyer J, Engdahl B, Johnsen E, Erbes C, Westermeyer J, et al. Post-traumatic stress disorder and service utilization in a sample of service members from Iraq and Afghanistan. Military Medicine. 2007 Apr;172(4):359-63.

74. Karney B, Ramchand R, Osilla K, Caldarone L, Burns R. Predicting the immediate and long-term consequences of Post-Traumatic Stress Disorder, depression and traumatic brain injury in veterans of Operation Enduring Freedom and Operation Iraqi Freedom. In: Tanielian T, Jaycox L, editors. Invisible wounds of war: psychological and cognitive injuries, their cosequences, and services to assist recovery. Santa Monica, CA: Rand Corporation; 2008. p. 119-66.

75. Rosenheck R, Leda C, Gallup P. Combat stress, psychosocial adjustment, and service use among homeless Vietnam veterans. Hosp Community Psychiatry. 1992 Feb;43(2):145-9.

76. Kasprow WJ, Rosenheck R. Substance use and psychiatric problems of homeless Native American veterans. Psychiatr Serv. 1998 Mar;49(3):345-50.

77. Leda C, Rosenheck R, Gallup P. Mental illness among homeless female veterans. Hosp Community Psychiatry. 1992 Oct;43(10):1026-8.

78. Benda BB. Survival analyses of social support and trauma among homeless male and female veterans who abuse substances. Am J Orthopsychiatry. 2006 Jan;76(1):70-9.

79. Report of the Defense Task Force of Sexual Assault in the Military Services | National Sexual Violence Resource Center (NSVRC): U.S. Department of Defense. 2009.

80. Hankin CS, Skinner KM, Sullivan LM, Miller DR, Frayne S, Tripp TJ. Prevalence of depressive and alcohol abuse symptoms among women VA outpatients who report experiencing sexual assault while in the military. Journal of Traumatic Stress. [Research Support, U.S. Gov't, Non-P.H.S.]. 1999 Oct;12(4):601-12.

81. Murdoch M, Nichol KL. Women veterans' experiences with domestic violence and with sexual harassment while in the military. Arch Fam Med. 1995 May;4(5):411-8.

82. Kimerling R, Street AE, Pavao J, Smith MW, Cronkite RC, Holmes TH, et al. Military-related sexual trauma among Veterans Health Administration patients returning from Afghanistan and Iraq. American Journal of Public Health. [Research Support, U.S. Gov't, Non-P.H.S.]. 2010 Aug;100(8):1409-12.

83. Suffoletta-Maierle S, Grubaugh A, Magrude K, Monnier J, Frueh B. Trauma-related mental health needs and service utilization among female veterans. J Psychiatr Pract. 2003;9(5):367-75.

84. Noonan ME, Mumola CJ. Veterans in State and Federal Prison, 2004. Washington, DC: US Department of Justice, Office of Justice Programs, Bureau of Justice Statistics. 2007.

85. Rosenheck RA, Banks S, Pandiani J, Hoff R. Bed closures and incarceration rates among users of Veterans Affairs mental health services. Psychiatric Services (Washington, DC). 2000;51(10):1282-7.

86. Greenberg G, Rosenheck R. Mental Health and Other Risk Factors for Jail Incarceration Among Male Veterans. Psychiatric Quarterly. [10.1007/s11126-009-9092-8]. 2009;80(1):41-53.

87. Black DW, Carney CP, Peloso PM, Woolson RF, Letuchy E, Doebbeling BN. Incarceration and veterans of the first Gulf War. Military Medicine. 2005;170(7):612-8.

88. Erickson SK, Rosenheck RA, Trestman RL, Ford JD, Desai RA. Risk of incarceration between cohorts of veterans with and without mental illness discharged from inpatient units. Psychiatric Services (Washington, DC). [10.1176/appi.ps.59.2.178]. 2008;59(2):178-83.

89. McGuire J, Rosenheck RA, Kasprow WJ. Health status, service use, and costs among veterans receiving outreach services in jail or community settings. Psychiatr Serv. 2003 Feb;54(2):201-7.

90. Metraux S, Caterina R, Cho R. Incarceration and homelessness. Stephen Metraux. 2008:1-.

91. Samuels P, Mukamal D. After Prison: Roadblocks to Reentry: Legal Action Center2004.

92. Pearson J, Davis L. Serving parents who leave prison: final report on the work and family center. Denver, Colorado: Center for Policy Research. 2001.

93. Thoennes N. Child support profile: Massachusetts incarcerated and paroled parents. Denver, Colorado: Center for Policy Research. 2002.

94. Benda BB, Rodell DE, Rodell L. Crime among homeless military veterans who abuse substances. Psychiatr Rehabil J. 2003 Spring;26(4):332-45.

95. Copeland LA, Miller AL, Welsh DE, McCarthy JF, Zeber JE, Kilbourne AM. Clinical and demographic factors associated with homelessness and incarceration among VA patients with bipolar disorder. Am J Public Health. 2009 May;99(5):871-7.

96. Stovall JG, Cloninger L, Appleby L. Identifying homeless mentally ill veterans in jail: a preliminary report. J Am Acad Psychiatry Law. 1997;25(3):311-5.

97. Steadman HJ, Barbera SS, Dennis DL. A National Survey of Jail Diversion Programs for Mentally Ill Detainees. Hosp Community Psychiatry. 1994;45(11):1109-13.

98. Broner N, Lattimore PK, Cowell AJ, Schlenger WE. Effects of diversion on adults with co-occurring mental illness and substance use: outcomes from a national multi-site study. Behavioral Sciences & the Law. [Article]. 2004;22(4):519-41.

99. Case B, Steadman HJ, Dupuis SA, Morris LS. Who succeeds in jail diversion programs for persons with mental illness? A multi-site study. Behavioral Sciences & the Law. [10.1002/bsl.883]. 2009;27(5):661-74.

100. Shafer MS, Arthur B, Franczak MJ. An analysis of post-booking jail diversion programming for persons with co-occurring disorders. Behavioral Sciences & the Law. [10.1002/bsl.603]. 2004;22(6):771-85.

101. Sirotich F. The Criminal Justice Outcomes of Jail Diversion Programs for Persons With Mental Illness: A Review of the Evidence. J Am Acad Psychiatry Law. 2009;37(4):461-72.

102. Steadman HJ, Cocozza JJ, Veysey BM. Comparing outcomes for diverted and nondiverted jail detainees with mental illnesses. Law and Human Behavior. 1999;23(6):615-27.

103. Steadman HJ, Naples M. Assessing the effectiveness of jail diversion programs for persons with serious mental illness and co-occurring substance use disorders. Behavioral Sciences & the Law. 2005;23(2):163-70.

104. Wilson DB, Mitchell O, MacKenzie DL. A systematic review of drug court effects on recidivism. Journal of Experimental Criminology. 2006;2(4):459-87.

105. 105. Toomey S. Diversion program for vets is offered. Anchorage Daily News. July 14, 2004.

106. Russell RT. Veterans Treatment Court: A Proactive Approach. New England Journal on Criminal and Civil Confinement. 2009;35:357-.

107. Hawkins JMD. Coming Home: Accommodating the Special Needs of Military Veterans to the Criminal Justice System. Ohio St J Crim L. 2010;7:563-849.

108. Under Secretary for H. Information and recommendations for services provided by VHA facilities to Veterans in the criminal justice system. 2009.

109. Moral Waivers and the Military. The New York Times. 2007.

110. Schmitt E. Its Recruitment Goals Pressing, the Army Will Ease Some Standards. New York Times. 2004.

APPENDIX A. PEER REVIEW COMMENTS/AUTHOR RESPONSES

PEER REVIEW COMMENTS - Epidemiological evidence regarding homelessness among Veterans

Reviewer No.	Comment	Response
Question 1:	***Are the objectives, scope, and methods for this review clearly described?***	
1	Yes.	
1	Comments: The numbers and letters used in the research objectives are distracting. I would use 1-4 and then use bullets for the sub questions.	We have revised the format of the document to comply with the standard VA Evidence-based Synthesis Program (ESP) style template. We think this should address the concerns of the reviewer.
1	In addition, the methods section should precede the discussion on the structural causes of homelessness.	This has been corrected in a way that follows the template of the ESP program.
1	The description of data sources could benefit from elaboration on limitations and that the limitations of the current research are a laundry list – are there key issues that you could group?	We have added a more detailed section describing the limitations of the datasets and hope that this addresses the concerns of the reviewer.
2	Yes.	
2	Very well-defined research questions.	
3	Yes.	
3	The key questions defined are very cogent and relevant to the current policy issues and priorities facing VA. The evidence synthesis reflects a tremendous amount of work and the authors should be commended.	
3	The conceptual model developed as part of this paper is nicely conceived and constructed and I feel it could be more prominently represented in the paper as (1) a means of organizing the data (2) a contextualizing in greater detail of the intermediate and mediating roles postulated in the paper. Toward both of these objectives, the schematic could be streamlined somewhat to more clearly define these relational dynamics.	We thank the reviewer for their comments on the Conceptual Model. We have modified the model and hope that the relationships are easier to follow. We've also relocated the Figure and discussion of the model and hope that it acts, as the reviewer suggests, as a frame for organizing the subsequent discussion of the topic.
4	It was very comprehensive.	
Question 2:	***Is there any indication of bias in our synthesis of the evidence?***	
1	No.	
1	The paper is balanced and fair.	
2	No.	
2	For the most part no- see comment 4.4 below.	
3	Yes - limited	

Reviewer No.	Comment	Response
3	The biggest problem and challenge with this synthesis is that for much of the research on homeless persons and homeless Veterans, there are inconsistent definitions, metrics for assessment, and methodologic rigor assigned to sampling, unmeasured population dynamics, geographic biases, etc. You do a very nice job of describing this at the beginning of the paper but it needs to be more prominently factored into some of the conclusions presented in the body of the paper. An example of this is in the discussion about social support and its role in homelessness, combat exposure, etc. There are objective measures of social and social support networks (we used the Rand Social Support Network Survey in our studies) that have been highly correlated with several features of homelessness. The surrogate measure of marital status is far weaker, nontemporal, and without any validation that I am aware of – I am concerned about any conclusions being drawn off that metric. Similarly, as you have noted, homeless research on substance use and abuse has historically been challenged by inconsistencies in how use is measured, whether it reflects current use while homeless or pre-homeless (and more likely contributant use). There are also definite distinctions between hazardous use, abuse, and dependence and its impact on functioning, risk, and capacity to engage in services. Knowing which studies employed any of the Addiction Severity index modules in making their determinations would be helpful in considering the rigor of the data being presented. Greater attention to this level of detail is needed in the synthesis. This is an area where you may find expanding the search beyond homeless veterans to homelessness in the general population will be of help. The only other concern that needs to be addressed is the age of some of the data – inferences drawn from data that are now 20-25 years old may not be relevant to the dynamics of homelessness today.	Corrected. We have included a more direct discussion describing the inconsistencies that we found among the various studies that examine the prevalence of substance abuse or mental illness among homeless Veterans. We have also identified additional measures that might provide better insights into issues of social support and social capital.

Question 3:	Are there any studies on the epidemiology of homelessness among Veterans that we have overlooked?	
1	No.	
1	This review is one of the most comprehensive that I've read.	
2	No.	
2	Very thorough assessment of the literature and innovative use of emerging search programs	
3	Yes - limited	
3	The challenge for the team to consider is whether it is better to take well-constructed and methodologically rigorous studies about homelessness in the general population and apply them to homeless Veterans over what are sometimes less well constructed or significantly biased data (in terms of selection bias, validity/reliability of findings, etc.) that is specific to homeless Veterans. Many of papers specific to homeless veterans are drawn from samples of veterans enrolled in VA programs or services for homeless persons and reflect a level of engagement, support and capacity that may not be reflective of the overall population of homeless veterans – most of whom do not get there care in the VA. This is particularly relevant when causality or dimensional relationships are being inferred or considered.	Because of the exploratory nature of this review, and because the purpose of the report was to provide background on what's known about homelessness among Veterans, we felt it better addressed the goals of the report to identify and report on studies specifically about Veterans and to discuss the limitations of those studies. We supplemented this with a brief background discussion of the literature on homelessness more broadly and hope that this report will prove useful in identifying the need for more methodologically rigorous and broadly applicable studies about homelessness among Veterans.

Reviewer No.	Comment	Response
4	My only concern is that the substance abuse prevalence section is a little light, I believe more literature exists. Also, the reference was from an older study. For example O'Connell, Kasprow, Rosenheck, 2010 report on HUD VASH client demographics and include data on substance abuse. Also, Rosenheck fairly frequently reports this data as well in his studies.	We have revised our discussion of the substance abuse issues and hope that it addresses the concerns of the reviewer.

Question 4: *Please write additional suggestions or comments below. If applicable, please indicate the page and line numbers from the draft report.*

Reviewer No.	Comment	Response
5	Page 3, Question 1a: Report states Veterans are 2x the risk of homelessness compared to the general population. Need to clarify comparison as children should not be included in denominator. Also, since men are more likely to be homeless (not just Veterans), comprising almost two-thirds of all homeless adults, it is important to factor this into comparisons. Without these adjustments it appears veteran status alone places individuals as far greater risk.	We have added language to address the reviewers comment.
5	Page 4, Question 2b: Homeless Veterans are more likely to be African-American. This is not addressed.	We have included additional language addressing the over-representation of Blacks among the homeless and of the over-representation of Veterans, both Black and White among the homeless.
5	Page 7: When discussing the minimum wage the paper uses 2004 as a reference point to describe the impact of its declining value; however, the minimum wage was increased after that date. This makes the selection of 2004 appear to be used to bias the conclusion. Also, 14 states have minimum wages higher than the federal minimum wage. It may be more effective to describe the declining value of the minimum wage in relation to the increasing FMR of apartments.	We have edited the text to provide a more general description of the declining value of the minimum wage in relation to the cost of housing.
5	Page 12 (bottom), Question 1b: Paper states Veterans are more likely to be unsheltered than other groups. AHAR does not state this as factual, only speculates that this is a possibility.	We have revised the language to indicate the speculative nature of this perspective.
5	Page 13, Question 1b: "Kuhn reports 24% increase in homeless families". Need to clarify statement as it leads the reader to incorrectly conclude that this is the increase in overall family homelessness. This increase only reflects what VA staff report they have seen *at their facilities*.	We have revised the language here to be clearer that we are reporting on an increase in staff reports of increases in people seeking services.
5	Page 24, Incarceration: No mention is made on the impact of child support. Legal assistance for child support is ranked as the second highest unmet need in the CHALENG report. Unpaid and unaffordable child support obligations often act as a significant barrier to a Veteran's ability to resume independent community living. This burden is particularly acute among ex-offenders. The typical incarcerated parent owes $20,000 in child support when released from prison, with payment schedules averaging $225 to $300 per month (Center for Law and Social Policy, 2008). Minimum wage workers have little hope of making these payments while supporting themselves. Unresolved child support debts can result in liens against bank accounts, denial of credit, inability to secure a lease, failure in background checks commonly a part of job applications, forfeiture of driver's licenses, and ultimately re-arrest.	We have expanded this section to address the issue of child support and thank the reviewer for their very helpful comment.

Reviewer No.	Comment	Response
5 (cont.)	As child support payments are deducted automatically from paychecks, workers often quit once their pay is garnished, returning to the underground economy to avoid child support. For ex-offenders, participation in the underground economy often means a return to illegal activity (Center for Law and Social Policy, 2007). Hence, legal assistance around the issue of child support is one key to helping Veterans meet their obligations to society, while still having the means to avoid relapsing to homelessness.	
1	The manuscript needs a thorough copy edit.	We agree and have done so.
1	On page 9, please expand on the limitations of each data source.	We have added a more detailed section describing the limitations of the datasets and hope that this addresses the concerns of the reviewer.
1	Page 10: this is a laundry list and the narrative doesn't flow. Is there a better structure? Perhaps grouping?	We agree that this section needed better organization. We have reorganized so that similar topics are addressed together, and, as suggested by the reviewer have added subheads to make clear how the topics are grouped together.
1	Page 11. Second paragraph: double check the definition. I think the first line is inaccurate. McKinney-Vento does include those living in transitional housing as homeless.	We checked Perl (2009) and the McKinney-Vento Act. No change to our statement is needed. Currently, only those living in transitional housing for the mentally ill are included. The Hearth Act will add others living in transitional housing to the definition of homelessness.

Reviewer No.	Comment	Response
General Comments		
6	I have two serious problems with your conceptual model: First, you group PTSD and Mental Illness together, in the center of the model, and directly associate them with homelessness (giving the association a strong arrow and two asterisks, which are the strongest form of association you have in the model). This contradicts what you state in several places in your report, where you say there is a lack of evidence directly relating PTSD and homelessness (e.g., pps 29 and 33). The problem here, obviously, is that MI and PTSD should not be coupled like this. MI is of course a catchall term and PTSD is a specific diagnosis. Associations with MI in general should best be broken down into more specific components. Even severe mental illness (which typically includes only schizophrenia and major affective disorders) is a better designation than just MI. And PTSD should have its own box, which, according to the evidence you review, should NOT have a direct association with homelessness. Including the model as it is would be seriously problematic, as it would in effect create a PTSD-Homelessness link that future research could use cite from this review. Second, alcohol and substance abuse have only weak, indirect associations with homelessness in the model. This would contradict your text, where on p 28 you cite, among others, a Wenzel study and a Winkleby et al. study as finding such associations. It also runs counter to a broad range of research among non-Veterans who make this SA-homelessness association. If you mean to disassociate homelessness and SA, as you effectively do in the model (and invite others to cite you), then you need to insert specific text in the report that explicitly explains your decision to do this.	1) We thank the reviewer for sharing these concerns. Further discussion led to a substantial revision of the model for overall clarity. We dropped the use of the more general term "mental illness." "Underlying psychiatric illness" was added to a box labeled "shared early life exposures," since the strongest evidence on this issue for a homeless veteran population comes from Rosenheck and Fontana 1994, which used psychiatric treatment before age 18 as a variable. As our reports notes, it is unfortunate that few studies involving homeless veterans actually assess for schizophrenia, unless they are among individuals seeking treatment for mental illness, in which case the sampling frame raises serious issues for the generalizability of any associations found. There is now a box labeled "PTSD/Depression/Anxiety." While frequent comorbidity might provide justification for this cluster, our model groups these conditions together because a) the veteran-specific evidence cited (Washington and Yano 2010) also groups PTSD and anxiety disorders together, and b) because the general homelessness literature cited finds associations between depression and homelessness (as well as psychiatric disorders). Our report states that "the evidence linking PTSD to homelessness remains limited by the small number, small size and/or non-generalizable sampling methods of existing studies." This is not the same thing as stating that there is no evidence, and we stand by the model's representation of an association between PTSD/Depression/Anxiety and homelessness. Here as elsewhere in the revised model, we have added a black box along the association pathway to indicate that the mechanism for the association is poorly understood. We hope this will encourage users of our model to direct future efforts towards understanding mediating factors. 2) We thank the reviewer for pointing out the discrepancy between the research that we site describing the association between substance abuse and homelessness and the weak link presented in the conceptual model. We have revised the model to indicate that substance abuse has a strong association with homelessness, but that the path through which substance abuse effects the risk of homelessness remains unknown. We also note in the text that evidence for substance abuse as a causal factor for homelessness has been inconsistent. Much of the research on substance abuse and homelessness employs a cross-sectional sampling frame, and thus, cannot demonstrate cause and effect. We discuss the limitations of studies examining substance abuse and homelessness in detail in our "Assessing the Limitations of the Current Research" section.

Reviewer No.	Comment	Response
6	Your review of the CHALENGE and AHAR counts should do more to look at the methodological problems involved in the estimates. CHALENGE, as you say, has traditionally relied at least partly on expert assessments, which (as you never point out) is a notoriously inaccurate means to assess homeless population size (plenty of cites available on this) and biases towards overcount. This is not a slam on CHALENGE but a recognition that they were doing their best with the limited data that was available and that the report primarily seeks to examine needs and needs fulfillment among the homeless Vet population. AHAR on the other hand, due to their reliance on mainstream homeless services data, is biased towards undercount. This leaves, as you point out on 22, a substantial gap (52,000 to 107,000) in the Vet estimates which, instead of examining further, you sidestep by only saying both numbers address the "seriousness of the problem." As I said earlier, the Vet-AHAR bridges these two methodologies, both in its estimate and in its methodology, and needs to be included here. One other note here, in your stating the overrepresentation of risk for homelessness among Veterans, you need to distinguish between studies such as were done by Rosenheck and his colleagues that sex and age adjust the populations to get a more accurate representation of risk, and other studies that don't.	We have expanded on the discussion in this section and have included a discussion of the recently released Veteran AHAR along with data from that report. However, we feel that we adequately discussed the methodological problems of the CHALENG and AHAR counts along with the strengths and weaknesses of the epidemiology of the homeless more generally. We understand the reviewer to be referring to the study by Rosenheck and Frishman (1994) of Vietnam-era Veterans that suggested that over-representation was attributable to disproportionate numbers of Veterans in the youngest cohorts (age 20-34) of homeless White males, and the follow-up study by Gamache and colleagues (2001). We do not disagree with the reviewer about this. However, we are suggesting that, for the reasons discussed in the section on Assessing the Limitations of Current Research, more work needs to be done to understand why Veterans are over-represented.
6	On 28-29, you state question #2a but don't put any text to answer it. This is confusing, and the reader might assume, but cannot be sure, that this question is answered in the text to 2b. Why not combine these questions, then, or at least signal somewhere that 2a is answered in 2b	We agree, this was confusing and have combined the questions as suggested by the reviewer.
6	On page 29, you mention that there appear to be "unique, military related pathways by which Veterans acquire these risks [for homelessness]" yet there are NO specifics, and NO citations, to specific pathways either in the response to Question #2b or in the response to Question #3, the section in which the author states these pathways will be taken up in more detail, beyond a weak finding by Rosenheck and colleagues between heavy combat and homelessness. The omission in offering up specific evidence to back up this assertion, considering this is a "Best Evidence Synthesis" is very surprising.	The concept of a pathway, as used in our report, is crucially different from a direct association. Given that the existing evidence does not find that Veterans differ substantially from non-Veterans in terms of the risk factors most strongly associated with homelessness in general, it is important to try to understand what, if anything, is qualitatively different about Veterans' experiences that might increase their risk of these shared or common exposures. The conceptual model was revised to clarify how military specific exposures are associated with a number of other exposures that are in turn shared with the general population; these shared exposures are more often directly associated with homelessness, but the influence of military-specific exposures on the prevalence or severity of shared exposures may be significant. These chains of exposures are the pathways referenced. The discussion of these issues has been expanded under the section describing the evolution of the conceptual model on pages 13-14. More generally the section devoted to answering Key Question 3 is structured to explore the evidence for these pathways, which, as the report suggests, might include the specific salience, in a Veteran population, for examining military sexual trauma and/or combat exposure as precursors to PTSD/Anxiety/Depression, or post-deployment readjustment difficulties leading to low income.

APPENDIX B. TECHNICAL EXPERTS CONSULTED AND REVIEWERS

TECHNICAL EXPERTS CONSULTED

Ted Amann
Director of Homeless Programs
Central City Concern
Portland, Oregon

Monica Beemer
Executive Director
Sisters of the Road
Portland, Oregon

Lillian Gelberg, M.D., MSPH
Professor of Family Medicine
UCLA Geffen School of Medicine
Los Angeles, California

Don Miller
Chief Counsel
Housing and Urban Development
Portland, Oregon

Fran Randolph
Director of the Division of Services and Systems Improvement
SAMHSA, Center for Mental Health Services

Jim Reuler, M.D.
Professor, Department of Medicine
Oregon Health and Science University
Portland, Oregon

Robert Rosenheck, M.D.
Director, Northeast Program Evaluation Center and
Professor of Psychiatry and Public Health
Yale University School of Medicine
New Haven, Connecticut

Annetta C. Smith
Population Division
U.S. Census Bureau

REVIEWERS

Mary K. Cunningham
Senior Research Associate
Urban Institute

Amy Kilbourne, Ph.D., MPH
VA Serious Mental Illness Treatment Resource and Evaluation Center

John Kuhn
National CHALENG Coordinator

Stephen Metraux, Ph.D.
National Center for Homelessness Among Veterans

Thomas O'Toole, M.D.
Providence VA Medical Center

David Smelson, Psy.D.
Bedford VA Medical Center

www.ingramcontent.com/pod-product-compliance
Lightning Source LLC
Chambersburg PA
CBHW081606170526
45166CB00009B/2852